COPYRIGHT, COVER DESIG

Nature's 9 Health Laws Break Them & Y ...me! Stay Out of
Jail. A How to Guide to Heal Your Body Naturally!

Copyright©2015 Dr. Megan Lebon ND

Cover by Warren Hutson[64]

**The information in this book represents the viewpoint and
experiences of the author. It is not intended to replace or supersede
medical advice from your physician. For this reason the
author/publisher is not responsible or liable for any injury or loss
incurred for any individuals who use the information presented in
the text to self-treat. Readers are encouraged to seek
recommendations from and be supervised by a qualified health
professional.**

Table of Contents

DEDICATION

I dedicate this book to YOU the reader! Maybe you do not have an official diagnosis but you feel tired and horrible! Maybe doctors told you that you have a certain disease and that you will have it forever. Do not believe that! Start learning and getting back in tune with Nature's 9 Health Laws and watch what your body will do! On the other hand, perhaps you are not sick and you just want to make sure you STAY healthy! Whether you are a boy or girl, whether you are a young/middle age/elder adult, whether you are fat or skinny, no matter what color you are or what nationality or religion you belong to...this book is to encourage, motivate and empower you to take your health and your life under control! HOORAY for natural healing!

ACKNOWLEDGEMENTS

I would like to thank **GOD** who is the author of my past, present and future! Thank you to my **beloved FAMILY** who have been the support and driving force for my entire life allowing me to achieve what I have! Thanks *especially my mom* who recently has been my right hand "woman" through the entire establishing of my office and with this writing process! Thanks to my dad for creative insights and for influential management; to my sister, brother and my sister-in-law, for their honest critique and who keep me laughing; to my nephews who inspire me with their brilliance; my Ori family; and to my favorite aunt in France M-A for a listening ear! Thanks also to my **best friends** from AAA, GSU and my SCNM IC...*especially my princess*! Special thanks to WH for technical support during the writing process! I also thank my friends in Georgia, my beloved PFS; my supporters from "Megan's Update" and my friends in Arizona *especially* my asparagus leaf for the motivation to write the book! Many thanks to you all! This would not have been possible without your well wishes, prayers and thoughts!

MY HEALTH STORY

I was born in Paris, France, my family immigrated to the U.S. in my childhood and I have always wanted to be a doctor since I was 10 years old! I studied science in university with the plan of becoming a conventional medical doctor. I was 24 years old and had just graduated from university and was planning to go to medical school in a foreign country when *BAM!* out of nowhere two weeks before I left, my body just started slowly swelling up with fluid. I ignored the symptoms and I left the U.S. anyway to start school in Cuba. Once I arrived, I never started school officially though because after two weeks I was urgently admitted to a hospital in Havana to stop a life-threatening situation of having my kidneys stop working. Fluid was building up everywhere in my body since I had stopped peeing. I had gained about 30 pounds in a few days from drinking water but not being able to pee! My eyelids and face were so swollen I did not recognize myself! My feet were too fat for shoes so I only wore flip-flops and I even had a pocket of space in my back that I called my "camel hump" from where fluid was gathering. My legs, stomach and even my bum got bigger! Fluid was everywhere! After being in the hospital a month to stabilize me, I was discharged and told to return to the United States for "conventional or standard" treatment for a serious lifelong and "incurable" disease that I had never heard of. I was shocked with my diagnosis because I had never been sick as a child or young adult! There were no sick people in my family either! It just seemed to come from nowhere!

Once I returned to the U.S. I went to see a specialist, we did lab work and of course ALL of the lab work was bad (in the "red") and the specialist then told me about all the side effects of the pharmaceutical drug treatments of which the most common side effects included: fatigue, hair loss, weight gain, osteoporosis, infertility, depressed immune system and leukemia. So essentially, I was told that I could become a 24-year-old tired, bald, fat, brittle boned, infertile, sickly and cancerous young woman! And that was just the common side effects of the FIRST drug they wanted me to use...not even to mention the second more powerful one! I just felt that the drug treatments would be kill me faster than the illness progression and was very depressed and afraid!

Unbeknownst to me, my father had been looking around for natural healing programs and found the one by Dr. Richard Shulze[4] (see his cleanse information in chapter 10) and I did that for 30 days. This program included all of the natural therapies, healing herbs and juices that allow the body to get rid of trash, take in nutrition and essentially get back in tune with Nature's 9 Health Laws—laws that I knew nothing about at the time. After doing the program, I redid my lab work and after only 30 days, all the bad lab values had moved into the "green" or improved...all except for two, which had still improved! I could not believe what a difference 30 days could make in my health! That pushed me to go into a naturopathic medical program since I am LIVING and HAVE LEARNED how to help the body restore health to itself!
I continue to utilize Nature's 9 Health Laws in my own life! You can learn and live this too with my book! So let us get started! ---*Dr. Megan*

INTRODUCTION

WRRR! RRR! Sirens! You look in the rearview mirror of your car and see the flashing blue lights of a police car telling you to pull over. *Oh no!* The policeman steps out and says "Did you know you were speeding?" and you respond **"No, I thought I was going the speed limit!"** He replies "You were going 15 miles over the speed limit, so I'm going to have to give you a ticket". To which you reply **"Please officer, I REALLY thought I was going the speed limit, the last time I looked I was within the limit!"** And he says "Well, you are above the posted speed limit *now* so here is your ticket!"

What is a LAW? It is a rule or set of rules that we must follow or else there will be consequences. Consider our driving laws: if we are speeding or run a red light, and we get stopped by the police—whether we knew that we were speeding or not/ whether we saw the light was red or not DOES NOT MATTER because the driving laws say that if we are driving a car, we should have already learned the road rules and be alert and follow them or else we will get in trouble! Now, if we are lucky, we may break the rules a few times without being caught, or if we are caught, the policeman may let us go without a ticket, but if we are consistently breaking the road laws we will have CONSEQUENCES: maybe we will cause an accident, get a traffic ticket, and even maybe get some JAIL TIME! Well did you know that NATURE has given us 9 HEALTH LAWS? And just like road laws, if we consistently break even one of them, we will cause long-term illness to develop! Short-term illnesses like colds and flus help develop the immune system, but LONG TERM ILLNESSES like high blood pressure, cancer and diabetes break down the entire body slowly over time and are devastating! But there is hope! LEARN how to get back in tune with all 9 Nature's Health Laws, especially by "Tidying up your Tummy", so that your body can strive to RESTORE FULL HEALTH to itself just by CONSISTENTLY doing all 9!
You can do this!

CHAPTER 1: I'm sick because I'm full of trash?!? What are Nature's 9 Health Laws?

Yep! If you have some illness that you have had for more than 6 weeks, like a few of these most common illnesses: Diabetes, High Blood Pressure or Cancer then your body is FULL of TRASH! Normally, our bodies are constantly trying to clean out trash and debris from our insides but sometimes the body can get overwhelmed with different life stressors that then pull us out of tune with Nature's 9 Health Laws. **By the way, I learn best by hearing analogies, and I think maybe you will too, so this book will be full of them…starting right now! Analogy:** *We all know monkeys LOVE bananas right? (Nod your head yes), well if we put a monkey into a room and throw only one banana in there to him, he will probably peel and eat the banana superfast right? But what if we throw in 5 bananas at a time and then 10 bananas at a time? After a while, he will not be able to keep up with peeling and eating the bananas at the speed he did with just the one banana. Plus the peels will start to pile up in the room and if we keep throwing in bananas at that rate, eventually he will get buried under peels and bananas! Poor monkey.* ☹ This is what happens in your body when it gets overwhelmed with life stressors. The bananas represent life stressors and the monkey represents your body's ability to heal itself.

Have you ever gotten a cut on the hand/leg—without knowing you cut yourself and then noticed the healing scab a few days later? That happened because the body has the ability to restore health to itself! So why doesn't it do so with serious illnesses like high blood pressure, cancer and diabetes? It is because life's many stressors have overwhelmed it and it loses that ability.

LIFE STRESSORS

(1) **Environmental stressors**---toxins--heavy metals, pesticides on foods, toxic household cleaners
(2) **Mental/Emotional stressors**—births/deaths, marriages/divorces, moving to another city/state/country, change of job/career.
(3) **Physical stressors**—car accidents, falls, a physical assault, surgeries or other trauma.
(4) **Unhealthy lifestyle habits**—poor nutrition, using recreational/street drugs, abusing alcohol, dehydration/not drinking enough water, long-term use of prescription medications, and high stress.
(5) **Infectious organisms "bugs"**—viruses, bacteria, fungi and parasites.

Some of the stressors we created ourselves—by making certain bad decisions, while other stressors were completely out of our control and imposed upon us by our environment—like genetics or what happened to us in childhood. *Therefore, **if we are out of balance** with Nature's 9 Health Laws **the question is not IF** we will develop a long term debilitating illness, **but <u>WHEN</u>** will we develop it!* Remember, with a LAW, it does not matter if you broke it knowingly or unknowingly—the consequences are the same! **Therefore the cause of ALL long-term illness, no matter what the name of the illness/diagnosis: is coming out of balance with Nature's 9 Health Laws!**

Therefore, if you get back in tune with Nature's 9 Health Laws by making consistent lifestyle adjustments—then your body will strive to restore FULL health to itself from any illness!
You can do this!

WHAT ARE NATURE'S 9 HEALTH LAWS?
I am glad you asked!
(1) Air
(2) Water
(3) Nutrition
(4) Sleep
(5) Movement/exercise
(6) Time in nature/outside (grounding)
(7) Positive mindset/spirituality
(8) Purpose
(9) FUN!

WHERE DID NATURE'S 9 COME FROM ANYWAY?

Nature. Duh! Sorry, I am a bit of a smart aleck ☹

CHAPTER 2: So all this trash is making my body parts not work well?

Yes, life stressors that we brought onto ourselves through bad decisions (bad nutrition, too much alcohol or smoking) or life stressors that were forced onto us by our environment (genetics, a hazardous job, or where we grew up) can STILL affect us MANY years later! Often patients are surprised to hear that if they were in a car accident 5 years ago that the consequences of that accident could STILL be affecting them now; or how the fact that they smoked for 10 years, but quit smoking 30 years ago still does not mean their lungs are ok now!

Analogy: think about a car. What if you get a hammer and start hitting the hammer onto the side of the car door as hard as you can for a long, long time, for hours or days...until you get tired and decide to stop...(seriously readers, please do not try this experiment at home ☺)....that would create a big dent into the car right? Well once you STOP hitting the car with the hammer, you stop making the dent deeper/bigger. But will that dent ever just magically disappear? No right? To actually make the dent go away, you have to take the car to a mechanic and they have to do some SERIOUS bodywork to repair it. And if you have ever had damage to the side of your car, you know how even just a LITTLE dent can turn out to be a BIG problem and very expensive! ☹ Likewise in the body, just because you stopped drinking heavily years ago, or finally were able to change a job where you had to work under high stress conditions, that does not mean that right now, even many years later, that your body is not STILL hurting from those stressors. You know why? Because life does not stop! Life keeps on throwing things our way and if your body never got the chance to recover from the first insult... then it just continues to take hits while trying to fix itself as best as it can*!*

Analogy: did you ever play the game "dodgeball" when you were a kid? Basically, you are alone in the middle of the school yard or park and then your classmates/friends all have small rubber balls that they throw at you and your job is not to get hit by any of the balls. So if there is only one kid throwing the ball at you, you likely will never get hit. But if there are 2, 3 or 10 kids throwing balls at you the WHOLE time, you ARE going to get hit! And then all you can do is put up your hands and try to defend your head right? That is life! Our bodies are constantly hit 24/7 with pollution, stress, viruses etc. ALL the time!
The car dent is an example of how trash can build up over time with stressors. Unlike a car though, sometimes we are not able to restore a certain part(s) of the body to absolute full function if the damage is too great. However, most often if we get back in tune with Nature's 9 Health Laws and give the body parts the support that they need, we can help the body parts get rid of trash and restore health! ☺ **You can do this!**

CHAPTER 3: What are my body parts, how do they work and why should I care?

To properly take care of something, you HAVE to understand its purpose and the basic way it works or else you will not use it well! ***Analogy:*** *what if you saw a car, but did not know that its purpose is to move YOU from point A to point B and so instead of sitting inside the car and driving it, you get behind the car and YOU PUSH IT? That would be very silly...and heavy! Or what if you knew it was supposed to move you places but did not know what a gas tank is or that you have to put gas into it pretty often? So you just sit inside a car that has no gas! See how important it is to understand BOTH **(1)** the basic purpose and **(2)** what the basic operation of a car is?* Likewise your body's basic purpose is (1) to allow you to LIVE LIFE to the FULLEST, and your body's basic operation are (2) all of the organs/parts working together perfectly.

The best way to learn about your body parts and their function is to use many different analogies of things with which you are already familiar!

 BODY ANALOGY: your body is like a country*. So insert your name here: if it were me, my body would be the United States of Megan. You have a few regions-- the north, south, east and west. Think of each of your body's organs as cities so you have Heart city, Brain city, Lung city etc. Each city is composed of groups of neighborhoods, and the smallest unit in a neighborhood would be a cell or ONE house. Each cell/house has a lot of activity going on inside of it: packages and deliveries come into the house and trash and unused things are taken outside of the house. Each cell/house is responsible for producing items that its neighborhood, city and overall "United States of You" needs. We then transport all internally produced supplies like vitamins and minerals from our cells/houses to the other organs/cities or regions in the United States of You in semi-trucks/red blood cells which travel along your highways/blood vessels and also travel on the side roads/lymphatic system. We often use hormones/messengers in the United States of You to perform jobs and or deliver important information to your parts/cities. You can think of hormones/messengers as being like the mail carrier!*

BRAIN CITY/CENTRAL NERVOUS SYSTEM—*Analogy: The airport control tower of the United States of You!** Did you know that Hartsfield-Jackson Airport located in Atlanta, GA is currently the busiest airport in the world? It has more planes taking off and or landing and more passengers moving in and out of its walls than any other. Your brain is like the control tower at this airport! It must keep track of all events in and around your body, making sure that all planes/organs are working perfectly! It gathers information about events INSIDE your body in all of your* cities/organs *(just like keeping track of all the planes flying inside the United States of You)* as well as monitoring what happens OUTSIDE of your body *(planes that are flying into your airport from outside of the country).* The brain keeps track of all this info via long "wires" we call nerves.

The brain monitors information such as danger, heat/cold, your emotions, controls movements, just to name a few, and then makes decisions on things that need to change and then sends the orders for changes to be made in the cities/organs, muscles etc. in your affected body regions. ***Analogy:*** *You can also think of nerves as being like telephone poles, and the brain would be the actual telephone.* Since it is so important to make sure nothing is ever missed or else you will have your planes crashing to the ground, crashing into each other *(BAM!)* or maybe even foreign/enemy planes trying to sneak in to our airspace in the United States of You, the brain is ALWAYS on alert, even while you sleep! The administrative or 9am to 5pm working part of the brain turns off at night while you sleep so you can rest and rebuild, but the overnight watching part of the brain takes over then! The brain has two basic states of being: **(1) rest/relax**--like while you are eating, sleeping, or just sitting around, or **(2) fight/flight--**I should run away/am excited—like when you are exercising, scared/anxious, or angry.

HEART CITY/CARDIOVASCULAR SYSTEM—*Analogy: the Interstate/highway system of the United States of You!* *How do we get juicy Valencia oranges grown in Florida to New York? We can certainly fly them there of course, but we cannot buy oranges off the plane right? They have to get into grocery stores and how do they get there? Via the interstate or highways using semi-trucks!* That is Heart city's job, it sends out semi-trucks/red blood cells to make pickups and deliveries to all cities/organs and parts/muscles, fat etc. in the United States of You. These semi-trucks drive along your interstates/highways, which we call blood vessels or the circulatory system. You have highways/blood vessels that lead AWAY from Heart city called arteries and highways that return TO the heart called veins. Since the body's cities and counties ALWAYS need supplies these semi-trucks/red blood cells are always on the move constantly! Essentially, your heart has two phases, the time when it is sending out semi-trucks/red blood cells to all of your cities/organs/parts and then the time when it is receiving all the trucks returning from all your cities.

Analogy: *think of this action like a toilet—when you flush the toilet all the water leaves the toilet bowl. Then there is a brief time when the toilet bowl is refilling with water in preparation for the next flush.* The heart has four main sections: the top two sections receive trucks/blood from all cities and the bottom two sections send trucks/ blood away from the heart to all cities. When you think about a blood pressure reading the flushing part of the toilet is the same as when the heart is pushing out blood/the top number and the filling part is when the heart is receiving blood back into the heart/the bottom number. Heart city is a muscle and it **NEVER sleeps**. It works 24/7 and it only speeds up its beating—like when you exercise or are nervous (fight/flight mode) or it slows down like when you are eating or sleeping (relax/rest mode). The speed up/slowdown is controlled by Brain city based on the information Brain city receives about what is going on inside and outside the United States of You.

Unlike a toilet though, the heart is a closed system—meaning the same amount of semi-trucks/red blood cells that leave the heart must come back! *Thank goodness pee/ poop do not come back up into our toilets because that would be totally gross* ☹ Now the trucks do not all have to leave and return at the same time, but if they do not eventually leave and return in the **same day** then we have a problem that we call bleeding! *Analogy: think of a household with 2 parents, 2 kids and a dog. The parents and kids may each leave for work/school all at different times and even the dog may run around the neighborhood all day long, but at the end of the day if only 3 of the 4 people make it back home and the dog is also missing, then that is a problem!* **Note:** the body is constantly using the same semi-trucks/red blood cells over and over again, and then replacing old/broken down trucks with new trucks. The body loves to recycle in all of its parts and cities!

The three main reasons that semi-trucks/red blood cells do not make it back to Heart city in a timely manner is because of **(1)** blocked blood vessels/slow traffic **(2)** blood clots/accidents between trucks or **(3)** bleeding/trucks running off the road. We always want our highways to be moving fast and freely and any time we have **Scenario 1:** Blocked blood vessels-which can be caused by a poor diet-it is like having trash on the highway and then that will cause a slowdown in traffic *BEEP! HONK!* **Scenario 2:** If traffic was moving slowly and one truck did not see that another truck stopped, then the first truck runs into the second truck *RRRR! SMASH!* causing an accident/blood clot. A traffic jam or accident/blood clot in Brain city is called a stroke, a traffic jam or accident/blood clot in Heart city is called a heart attack!

Scenario 3: We can even have broken streets with big cracks in them/damaged blood vessels—caused by harmful substances such as tobacco, alcohol and street drugs and the bad quality highways/blood vessels can cause our semi-trucks to run completely off of the road/bleeding! So once Heart city does not have its necessary supply of semi-trucks/blood cells leaving and returning in a timely manner to feed its own city, as well as the other major cities in the United States of you like Lung city and Brain city then Heart city starts working poorly and we get SERIOUS and possibly LIFE THREATENING PROBLEMS! Any of the three scenarios above can make Heart city shut down/stop working and if Heart city stops YOU ARE DEAD!!! **If your heart does not start beating on its own or we**

cannot get the shock/defibrillator paddles onto you *(ZAP!)* then it is farewell, so long, adios, au revoir, game over, goodbye cruel world ☹

LYMPHATIC SYSTEM and LYMPH NODES—Analogy: the side roads and local police precincts. This system has two functions. **(1)** Sometimes, some trucks/red blood cells get off the main highways/blood vessels and travel along side roads so that they can make deliveries and pickups to your cities/organs, but then afterwards they must get back onto the main highways and go back to Heart city. This is the main function of the lymphatic system/side roads. **(2)** The second function is as part of your immune system. You can think of your lymph nodes as local police precincts all along your highway system...so that is where you will always find some police hanging out ready to catch any bad guys that speed by breaking the law in those areas!

You have police precincts/lymph nodes on the back of your head, sides of your face, under your jaw, running down both sides of your neck, running down your chest, in your under arms, all around your stomach and digestive organs, and along the inside of your legs. Apart from the police that stay at the local precinct, you also have police/white blood cells that are cruising along your highways/blood vessels—you will learn more about the patrol police in the Digestion city chapter. These lymph nodes are like little circles so when a policeman/white blood cell catches a bad guy like a virus or bacteria it may often get swollen and then it can feel like a little ball and may be tender to the touch. It is very common for the lymph nodes in your neck to swell and hurt when you have an infection and that is what we doctors are feeling for when we touch both sides of your neck!
*Note: Do not get the types of cells confused! Remember the **red** blood cells are our semi-truck drivers and **white** blood cells are our police officers!*

LUNGS CITY/RESPIRATORY SYSTEM---Did you know that air/oxygen is your body's #1 source of energy? So for ALL cities/organs and muscles in the United States of You we need a <u>**constant**</u> supply of it. Lung city's job is to take air/oxygen in from the outside/inspiration. At the same time, semi-trucks/red blood cells arrive from Heart city to load up on the new air that just came inside Lung city, so that they can deliver air to all the other cities/organs and areas of the body. For example, the semi-trucks/red blood cells deliver air to your leg muscles so that they can use it for energy to walk and run or to Brain city so that you can think! After you have used up the useful parts of air/oxygen, only trash remains, which we call carbon dioxide. Since we do not like trash in the body, at the same time that the semi-truck/red blood cells unload the useful air/oxygen at your leg muscles, they pick up the trash/carbon dioxide and put that into their trucks. Then they get back onto your highways/blood vessels, drive back to Lung city, and unload the trash/carbon dioxide there so that your lungs can breathe it out/exhalation!

THYROID GLAND COUNTY—*Analogy: it is like the Central Intelligence Agency (CIA) in the United States of You!* Its main role is to gather information and make changes in these main areas of your body: energy, body temperature (like being cold/hot), digestion, heart function, mood, and women's menstrual cycles. To do so, it makes a few thyroid hormones/messengers that will travel on your highways/circulatory system to go to Digestion city, Heart city, Brain city, and Reproduction city. *Wow! It does a lot! This little gland is small but mighty! When it is out of balance, you will have major problems!* It can either overwork (hyperthyroid) or underwork (hypothyroid). It has a very close working relationship with the Adrenal glands also.

DIGESTION CITIES/GASTROINTESTINAL SYSTEM: this is my area of specialization! *Analogy: this is Washington D.C.* Whatever happens here determines the state of health of the ENTIRE United States of You! It is the region that feeds all of your other cities/organs including Brain city and Heart city! Therefore, it requires its own chapter. But just for you to get a head start, the Digestive system is like a region in the United States of You because it has 5 organs/cities and 3 parts/counties: Mouth county, Esophagus county, Stomach city, Small Intestine city, Large Intestine/Colon city, Liver city, Gall Bladder county and Pancreas city. Read more about this MOST IMPORTANT region in the next chapter!

SPLEEN CITY: this city has two main functions. *Analogy function 1: this is the Pentagon in the United States of You! The pentagon is the headquarters of defense for the United States—the main branches of the military are the army and marines (on land), the navy (on sea), and the air force in the skies; and then of course we have the local police.* Now, most of the actual military is not at Spleen city because most of our "soldiers" are in Digestion city, however, there are a few "military bases" at the spleen and these soldiers train and develop their skills here. They set up "road blocks" for all semi-trucks/red blood cells that travel through Spleen city and check the drivers for bad guys such as viruses and bacteria or even cancer cells that may try to harm the United States of You! If the "soldiers" find any bad people, then they will arrest them and take them to jail or to be killed!

    Analogy function 2: this is your old semi-truck/red blood cell recycling center! The second function of Spleen city is to recycle old or broken down semi-trucks/red blood cells and use the recycled parts to make new trucks. The soldiers may take a "tire" from an old truck to put onto a new truck, or maybe a "windshield wiper" that is still useful. The body is very intelligent and recycles parts whenever it can, so that we do not have to waste energy to make new parts!

If a semi-truck/red blood cell is too damaged to use any of its parts in the recycling program then it will be completely destroyed/sent to the junkyard.

Note: Semi-trucks/red blood cells are NOT made in the spleen they are made inside Bone city inside Bone Marrow county, so the recycled parts from Spleen city are packaged into properly working semi-trucks/red blood cells and get back onto your highways/blood vessels and travel to your bones. You can read more about this in the Musculoskeletal city section.

KIDNEYS & BLADDER CITY/GENITOURINARY SYSTEM: Kidney city has **three main functions.** *Analogy function 1: the* **recycling center** *for* <u>nutrients/useful items</u> *in the United States of You.* Kidney city receives semi-trucks/red blood cells all day long, which are carrying useful items like calcium for strong teeth and bones, glucose/blood sugar for muscle energy and vitamins and minerals for hair and skin. The Kidney city workers will take these nutrients /useful items, keep some for use INSIDE Kidney city, and then recycle the rest of the nutrients by putting them back onto semi- trucks/red blood cells so they can get back onto your highways/blood vessels for use in all other cities.

     Function 2: helps **break down trash/harmful substances** that come into your body! Harmful substances include drugs (prescribed/over the counter or street/illicit), alcohol, soda, tobacco and environmental trash/toxins like pesticides. These harmful things come into your body get onto your highways/blood vessels and make their way down to Kidney city where the workers take them apart and then the bad items are sent to your bladder/holding tank—until your bladder is full and then the urine/liquid trash is flushed out to sea when you pee. *Hey, that rhymes! Get it? Sea…pee?* ☺

Note: Liver city is the main organ that breaks down MOST harmful things that come into the United States of You but Kidney city is the second one.

Tiny analogy: You can think of Liver city as the big metal detector in an airport which catches any BIG metal thing that comes through on you (as you walk through the scan) or in your suitcases as they roll through the machine. Kidney city then, would be like the metal detector WAND that the officials wave around you looking for smaller things…you understand the difference? Liver city does most of the big work. Read more about it in the Digestion city chapter!

     Function 3: *Kidney city is the* **water works department** *in the United States of you!* Its last main job is to help Heart city make sure your blood pressure stays stable…so if your blood pressure is too high or too low then Kidney city comes to the rescue! It does this by watching how many semi-trucks/red blood cells are coming through Kidney city per minute…if blood pressure is TOO HIGH then Kidney city will create "detours" on your highways/blood vessels to allow the roadways to clear up a little bit. Kidney city does this by making hormones/messengers that travel to Lung city to make these changes. On the other hand, if blood pressure is too LOW because you do not have enough semi-trucks/red blood cells on the roadways, then Kidney city will make different hormones/messengers and send them to Digestion city and then eventually to Bone Marrow county in Bone city, so that we can make more semi-trucks/red blood cells in order to keep our blood pressure stable. Understand? It is cool huh? ☺

ADRENAL GLANDS COUNTY—these two are like counties in the United States of You. Their **main job is to produce three different hormones/messengers that will travel all over your body** affecting mainly three functions: how your body handles **(1)** salt balance/blood pressure in the body—via Aldosterone hormone **(2)** stress & blood sugar—via Cortisol hormone **(3)** reproductive actions-via Estrogen and Testosterone hormones. *Note: most of the reproductive hormones are made in the Reproductive city but Adrenal county is second best.* Adrenal county is what gives you the energy (via cortisol hormone) to bounce out of bed first thing in the morning, ready to get your day started at school, work or wherever! When a person is under much stress, Adrenal county produces a lot of Cortisol/stress hormone and when this hormone stays high, it can really cause a lot of problems like super low energy/fatigue, belly fat and also problems in Digestion city! Adrenal Glands county and Thyroid Glands county work very closely together. If one of them is out of balance, it will pull the other out of balance too!
Analogy: think of a car. To start the car you need to turn the key in the ignition switch (that is the adrenal glands), but what keeps the car running once the car is already started is the engine (Thyroid gland). Make sense?

REPRODUCTION CITY/GYNECOLOGICAL SYSTEM: This **helps you be able to make your own little "mini-me"**! If we did not have this city/organ then there would be no more humans on the earth after we all died! There is a difference between what men/boys have in their city versus what women/girls have. Essentially, men have testes/the sperm holding room and then sperm/swimmers, while women have ovaries/the egg holding room, eggs/the future baby and a uterus/the baby hotel. Usually Reproductive city in boys and girls are like "ghost towns" with NO ACTION/ACTIVITY until puberty—which happens anytime between 10 years old to 14 years old for most boys and girls. Then at that time the United States of You will decide to send workers to these cities so that they can start working and the workers will make eggs start "hatching/maturing" in girls and start to make sperm in boys. Girls are actually already born with all the eggs that they will ever have and will start to lose an egg every month with their menstrual cycle/period. Once all the eggs are gone then that is when a woman will enter menopause/no more eggs time and she can no longer get pregnant. Men on the other hand, can make sperm from puberty almost until they die unless they have a medical problem that stops them from doing so. Did you know that a healthy sperm count in men has to be at least 20 million? So having more than 20 million is best. Wow! That is a lot of "swimmers" in mom's "pool" huh?

      Analogy: *To make a baby (babies do not come from storks!) the sperm have to swim (like fish!) out of the dad and into the mom from a very long distance through a sticky obstacle course to reach the 1 egg/future baby which is moving down from mom's ovaries/egg holding room. The sperm are trying to swim as fast as they can, racing down and bumping each other because only one can win at the finish line/the egg! Only the strongest swimmer will make it because this is such a long swim that it can take a couple of days! Once the winning sperm reaches the egg, then that first sperm and the egg stick together and NO other sperm can then join the party.* Now the egg and the sperm join together to become the baby. It travels down to mom's uterus/baby hotel and baby grows in mom's hotel for about 9 months or so until the United States of Mom decides that it is time to send the visiting baby out of her hotel and into the world!

BONES & MUSCLES CITY/MUSCULOSKELETAL SYSTEM: *Bone city* is responsible for giving you structure/a definite shape. Without bones, you would look like a seal! *I have nothing against seals—they are really cute, even though they are just big blobs.* In between two bones, we have joints/a space, where we usually have a gluey padding so that two bones do not rub together *(ouch!)* In Bone Marrow neighborhood, deep inside Bone city, is where we make: semi-trucks/red blood cells, the military and police/white blood cells, and road repair trucks/platelets— platelets are the first on the scene to try to repair a broken road/bleeding.

Muscle county is what allows us to move things in and around the United States of You. Did you know there are three different types of muscles? There is **(1)** the muscles that you can control by thinking—such as for moving arms and legs **(2)** muscles that you cannot control like the muscles in Digestion city that break apart your food and then **(3)** the muscles in Heart city that work ALL the time. The muscles that you can move are all over the United States of You and attach onto your bones. First, in Brain city you think about what you want to move—like your hand--and then a message is sent down from Brain city through the long wires/nerves and arrives at the "telephone pole" in hand muscle neighborhood and the nerve touches the muscle and tells him to move and then your hand moves! Another thing we should mention is that the body also has fat/cushion. *Fat county* is a backup energy source as well as a way to help keep the United States of You warm. When we get too much of this—usually through overeating--- we get...well, we get fat! ☹ Fat county is also where toxins/harmful things get stored when the body can't seem to get rid of them entirely. *Analogy: we do not want criminals running freely in the street/blood vessels because they can do harm* *right? Since we cannot get rid of them altogether we lock them up in jail (fat) until we can get rid of them later...at least in jail they are LESS of a threat to society!*

SKIN CITY/DERMATOLOGICAL SYSTEM: You may think that all Skin city does is to give us a color, but it actually does so much more! It has **four main functions**
(1) It is the #1 **defense system** for invaders that might try to "walk" into the United States of You! That is why cuts on the hands, legs etc. are usually healed very quickly so that no mean viruses or bacteria can crawl in!
(2) It keeps all your cities/organs and **parts inside**. Just imagine, without skin, your intestines at Digestion city would just be flopping around in the wind for everyone to see! *Yuck!*
(3) Helps to maintain a steady **body temperature**—not too hot, not too cold!
(4) Moves things in and out. The skin takes useful things from the *outside* of the United States of You inside so that we can use them, but it also helps get rid of harmful/bad things coming from deep *inside* the United States of You and puts them *outside*!

Most people when they see something like a bump or rash on the skin they think of it as being a "skin" problem...but actually, more often than not, a rash or skin reaction is your body trying to show you that there is a problem deeper inside the United States of You...and since you do not have X Ray vision to look deep inside yourself, your body will put a rash/bump out onto the skin so that you can see it and begin to look for the problem! In a small percent of cases rash/acne/skin problems will truly be because of having touched something like poison ivy, or a bad reaction to a lotion/product that you put onto your skin, but actually more often than not, the problem is coming from Digestion city!
Analogy: you are driving along the highway and then you come to a traffic jam and no cars can move anymore. You have stopped but you cannot actually see the cause of the traffic jam. That is because <u>the cause of the traffic jam is not where you stopped and where you can see, but it is</u> <u>actually miles away higher up!</u> Perhaps there is an accident, furniture that fell off a truck blocking a lane, or even a bunch of chickens crossing the road...ok, well maybe not the chickens crossing the road. It is kind of like that. Skin problems are usually not truly "skin problems" but a problem from far away deep within the body and very often in Digestion city.

TONSIL COUNTY and APPENDIX COUNTY: these are two tiny areas in the body but they are SO misunderstood and often extradited/cut out of the United States of You! ☹ Both of these counties are super important as a part of your defense system! *Tonsils county* are in the back of your throat and they are like a local police precinct that "checks" all the food and drink that comes inside so that you do not get any sneaky bacteria or viruses trying to come inside your country. When you cut out your tonsils then you lose one of the MAJOR FIRST local precincts that help fight invaders at one of the most common entry points! If the tonsils are inflamed it is because they have caught bad guys and this condition is usually not life threatening so it would be better to just call the rest of your body's defense/immune system (local police, army, navy, air force) to come to Mouth county to help fight the invaders!

Analogy: *cutting out tonsils is like getting rid of the border patrol police between Mexico, Canada and the U.S.*

Appendix County is another police precinct but it is in Digestion city at the beginning of Large Intestine/Colon city. In this case, if an invader has arrived into the United States of You and snuck past all of the police at the local precincts/lymph nodes along Mouth county and Digestion city, then when the "bad guy" gets to Large Intestine/Colon city the local police at Appendix county might catch him. **However, unlike Tonsils county, if Appendix county gets inflamed or infected, it can actually blow up and then that could become a life-threatening emergency if you do not get to the hospital right away!** The reason for that is Appendix county's location: it is in Large Intestine city where we have many helpful bacteria that help us with digestion and immune/defense function. If Appendix city becomes inflamed or infected and explodes that could release many of the bacteria from Large Intestine city and allow them to travel to other areas of the body where they will no longer be helpful but will cause harm!

Analogy: *When we allow prisoners to pick up trash along the highway, they are helpful for cleaning the streets right? However, if the prisoners manage to escape and leave the highway and go free into our neighborhoods—where they should not be--then they become very dangerous!* However, sadly there are many occasions when the appendix is removed, even when there is no sign of inflammation or that it will explode! In that case, do not remove it!

BODY PARTS LOCATION REVIEW! I could not find a picture I like. ☹ You look. ☺
- **Brain--in your head**
- Tonsils—at the back of your throat
- **Thyroid—in your neck**
- Heart—in the middle and left side of your chest between lungs, under ribs
- **Lungs—in your chest, under ribs**
- Liver and gallbladder—right side of body, partly under and below ribs
- **Stomach—below ribs, above belly button**
- Pancreas--below ribs, middle to left side of body
- **Spleen—below ribs, left side of body**
- Small Intestines--below ribs, in middle of body
- **Large Intestines/Colon—below ribs (*appendix is part of L.I. on the right side*)**
- Kidneys—one on right and left side of the body, in your back, below ribs.
- **Adrenals—one on top of the right and the left kidneys.**
- Bladder and Reproductive organs—all between your hips

BASIC LAB VALUES EXPLANATION!
What these common labs tell us about your health!

GENERAL:
- **Complete Blood Count and Comprehensive Metabolic Panel**—*information about Red Blood Cells, White Blood Cells, Liver, Kidney, Pancreas function and electrolyte levels (potassium etc.)*
- **Lipids**—*Cholesterol, HDL, LDL, Triglycerides--relates to heart health*

IRON:
- **Iron panel**—amount of iron available in your blood and how it is being used
- **Ferritin**—storage form of Iron--*shows inflammation and often liver disease*

BLOOD SUGAR:
- **Glucose**—level of blood sugar at a random time
- **Hemoglobin A1c**---indicates how high blood sugar levels have been for the past 3 months

THYROID: If we were using a car analogy the parenthesis () indicates the part of the car
- **TSH**—main hormone indicator of adequate thyroid function *(gas gauge)*
- **Free T3** —active form of thyroid hormone *(gas in the engine)*
- **Free T4**—storage form of thyroid hormone *(gas in gas tank)*
- **Reverse T3**--how well storage thyroid hormone is converting to active hormone *(leaking gas)*

HEART:
- **Homocysteine**--heart health and risk for bad heart event *(stroke, heart attack)*
- **hs-CRP (high sensitivity C reactive protein)**—inflammation and heart event risk

LIVER:
- **Hepatitis B and C titers**--indicates viruses that affect the Liver

HORMONES:
- **Adrenal glands**--Cortisol morning (AM) and evening (PM). *Highest in morning.*
- **Reproduction**-*Estrogen, Progesterone, Testosterone, DHEA*, PSA (for men only- prostate health).

IMAGING:
- **Electrocardiogram**—information about the electrical conduction of the heart
- **Echocardiogram**— the structure/muscles/pumping of heart
- **Chest radiograph**--gives a visual of the lungs and the heart
- **Upper endoscopy**—shows the throat, Stomach and first part of Small Intestine
- **Colonoscopy**—shows the Large intestine/Colon
- **DEXA/Bone scan-whole body**—shows all bones in body and their overall health

CHAPTER 4: Your digestive system-why ALL disease AND health begins here!
My specialty!

The Digestive System/Gastrointestinal system (GI) is the most important region—it is like Washington D.C. because it FEEDS the entire United States of you: Brain city, Heart city, Lungs city, Kidneys city, Reproduction city, Musculoskeletal city, Skin city, Spleen city, Thyroid and Adrenals counties! Just as ALL laws and all decisions that will affect the 50 states and all U.S. territories are determined in Washington D.C., through your GI region enters all of the many important nutrients needed to keep all other organs and parts functioning. Therefore, once this system is unbalanced it will quickly cause problems in one or multiple other organ systems! Inside this chapter you will learn:

- **GI Overview:** two Divisions--Digestion and Immune
- Purpose, function and parts of each division
- **Factors that can unbalance the GI**
- Common Symptoms and Diseases of each division
- **Other organs an unbalanced GI will affect**
- Common testing done to detect GI imbalances
- **How to rebalance support the GI**
- A photo of the GI

WHAT IS THE GASTROINTESTINAL SYSTEM (GI) MADE OF?
It has two divisions-the Digestive System and the Immune System. The Digestive System actually has **5 organs/cities** (Stomach city, Small Intestine city, Large Intestine/Colon city, Liver city, and Pancreas city and **3 parts/counties**: Mouth county, Esophagus county, Gall Bladder county. The Immune system division is mostly inside Large Intestine/Colon city.

WHAT IS THE PURPOSE OF THE DIGESTIVE AND IMMUNE SYSTEMS?
The digestive system's purpose is to break down a large piece of food that you can see (like an apple) and pull out from that apple microscopic elements that you cannot see like vitamins and minerals. The body can then use these nutrients in all your other organs/cities and parts/counties to keep the United States of You running smoothly. The immune system's/defense purpose is to protect (and often repair) your body from harm- from "bugs" that come from either inside/outside the United States of You--bad bugs like viruses, bacteria, fungi; or to protect you from toxins/harmful stuff like medications, drugs, alcohol, tobacco products and

heavy metals. Both divisions can also respond to other physical or emotional injuries.

HOW DO THE TWO DIVISIONS OF THE GI FUNCTION?
GI--Digestive Division
Mouth county-has teeth to break up big solid food into small liquid parts.
Esophagus county--a tube sending liquid food to Stomach city.
Stomach city--makes acid that further breaks apart liquid food; and the acid kills virus/bacteria on food that you eat too.
Liver city—does many things!
(1) Makes bile juice to help break up different types of foods: protein, carbohydrates and *especially* foods with fats in them.
(2) Breaks down Estrogens. Also breaks down toxins/harmful stuff from: foods, medications, illicit drugs, harmful chemicals and filters/cleans all things that come into the body via the mouth, before allowing them to entire blood circulation/highway/interstate
(3) Makes and breaks down cholesterol
(4) Makes special *proteins* used for many things such as: proteins to build your cells/houses; proteins to make cargo trucks to move items around; and antibodies that work in your police/immune system
(5) Stores and breaks down blood sugar for energy
(6) Helps make Vitamins K, A, D and E and also stores Vitamin B12 and the mineral called Iron. Whew! In case you did not catch it, Liver city does A LOT that will affect MANY areas around the United States of You!

Gall Bladder County--stores bile, the "juice" made at Liver city, a "juice" necessary for breaking up fatty foods for digestion. Since Liver city is SO busy, and does not know when you will eat, or how much you will eat, Liver city makes the necessary bile juice ahead of time and then stores it in Gall Bladder county so that the bile juice will be ready whenever you decide to eat. *Sadly, the removal of the gall bladder is far too common! It is very bad to take out your gall bladder just because it is not working well or because it has a few stones inside it.* **There is a dangerous situation where if a gallstone is blocking a duct/road leading from Gall Bladder county to Pancreas city, the bile duct road can explode and this is life threatening because it can cause bleeding.** However, if that is not your case meaning if you are not told that you need surgery IMMEDIATELY or else you will die and they actually have time to *schedule* your surgery in the next few weeks, then KEEP your Gall Bladder county and get back in tune with Natures 9!

Analogy: If your liver were like the engine of your car, the gall bladder would be the "gas tank" for the liver. QUESTION: would you cut out your gas tank from your car just because it was not working that well or because it had a few stones in it? No right? Because if you remove the gas tank you no longer have any way to store gas! Depending on the model and year of the car, you can no longer drive more than a few feet before you would have to add in more gas to your engine BY HAND! Most new car models will not work AT ALL without the gas tank. This would DRASTICALLY affect how far you are able to travel in your car. What a pain! Likewise, we cannot have proper digestion without bile juice made by Liver city and stored in Gall Bladder county. Improper digestion can lead to SERIOUS health problems including heart problems, digestive system diseases and cancer just to name a few.

Pancreas city--sends enzymes/workers to Small Intestine city that help further break up the food types: fats, protein, and carbs.

Small intestine city--looks at the liquid food flowing by, pulls out useful vitamins, minerals, blood sugar and more, and then loads them into the semi-trucks/red blood cells to be shipped via your highways/blood vessels to all your other cities that need those good things! *Analogy: imagine workers leaning over a conveyor belt, pulling things off, and leaving some things on that we do not need.*

Large intestine/Colon city-This city holds all non-useful food/trash/harmful stuff that came down from Small Intestine city and once full, you have a bowel movement and the solid trash is flushed out to sea! Large intestines also are full of bacteria that both work in your digestion as well as in your immune system/police.

GI—the Immune Division/Defense

This is the internal defense "Army/Navy/Air force/local police" of the United States of You! These are essentially billions of friendly bacteria and their main "precinct/base" is inside Large Intestine/Colon city but some of them also travel in your highways/blood vessels to "go out on patrol". This division is able to recognize what things inside your body are "you" like your own other organs/cities and parts/counties and what is not "you" or something that came from outside. They can determine whether to "chase/attack" something that came from outside (like a virus or bacteria) or to leave it alone because it could be useful like food. Some immune cells/defense teams attack anything that looks suspicious and kill it right away but do not remember the bad guy. While other immune cells "remember" the offending invader so that when they see it again they can attack even faster. If your defense team cannot kill/rid your body of the problem then they will store it in fat county "take it to jail". Your immune cells are called to any site of injury in your body too, like if you bump and bruise your toe, or have any kind of illness.

WHAT FACTORS CAN UNBALANCE THE GI?
Many factors can individually or collectively make your GI not work well:

- **Medications** (prescription or over the counter)—antibiotics, steroids, and antacids are the worst! *Read more about these three in chapter 13!*
- **Illegal/illicit street drugs** (cocaine, heroin etc.)
- Alcohol and Tobacco products
- **Gland/Hormonal imbalances:** especially Thyroid and Adrenal gland hormones
- **Nutritional deficiencies**: such as low iron or low vitamin B12
- **Nutritional excesses:** #1 high intake of processed sugars (soda, sweets, other sugar sources) #2 high salt intake from prepared foods like from restaurants, frozen, packaged or canned foods
- **Mental/Emotional stressors**
- Physical stressors (surgeries, car accidents, falls, or other physical trauma)
- **Environmental stressors** (heavy metals, pesticides, pollution)
- Infectious agents (virus, bacteria, fungi)
- **Genetic influences**

COMMON SYMPTOMS AND CONDITIONS OF THE DIGESTION DIVISION
If you have any of these symptoms occurring more than once a day, and or more than once a week then it is a persistent issue. *Something is not working well with your "Hole in the Middle"!* I call it the "hole" because anything you ingest whether food, supplements/prescribed medications goes in your mouth but may fall out the other end of your body without getting where it needs to go, if this system is not working well! Because until the item is properly packaged and put into your highway system/blood vessels it cannot be used by the United States of You! We have to tidy up your tummy!

Common Digestion Symptoms: Nausea, vomiting, bloating, gas, burping, diarrhea, constipation, alternating diarrhea/constipation, heartburn, indigestion, abdominal pain, difficulty swallowing, hernias, jaundice (yellow eyes, skin or nail beds), hemorrhoids, blood or mucus in stool/poop, food sensitivities, increase/decrease in appetite.

NOTE: *optimal pooping means 1 well-formed bowel movement (BM) after every meal you eat without straining—stool should be soft—no big hard planks or small hard rabbit pellets! ☺ Mediocre bowel function is MINIMUM one daily BM without straining and soft. If you are not going daily, or if you are going daily but straining, you are constipated and that is <u>the worst GI symptom</u> of all because it means trash/toxins are not being emptied properly from the United States of You! ☹ ☹*

Common Digestion Conditions: Esophagitis (inflammation of esophagus); **Gastritis/Gastroenteritis** (stomach and or small intestine inflammation…infection is also possible); **Acid reflux**; Gastro Esophageal Reflux Disease (GERD); Stomach or Intestinal **Ulcers; Cancers; Irritable Bowel Diseases (IBD)** like Chron's and Ulcerative Colitis; **Diverticulitis and Diverticulosis** (Large intestine inflammation and pouches/little "bags", respectively); **Cholecystitis and Cholelithiasis** (gall bladder inflammation and gall stones, respectively); **Pancreatitis** (inflammation of pancreas), **Celiac Disease** (small intestine cannot break down gluten protein); **Hepatitis** (inflammation of liver); **Cirrhosis** (a really sick, badly working liver), **High/Low Cholesterol** and **Diabetes**.

COMMON SYMPTOMS AND CONDITIONS OF THE IMMUNE DIVISION

When the immune division begins to function *less* than it should, we typically see an increase in infections: colds, flus or even long-term infections like viral or bacterial hepatitis. When the immune division becomes *more active* than it should we often see it attacking things it should not attack (like your own body parts instead of outside viruses or bacteria) and we call this autoimmunity.

Analogy: This is the same as "friendly fire" so it is like one of your policemen shooting another policeman instead of shooting the bad guy.

Common Immune Symptoms: fatigue; muscle weakness or pain; joint pain or swelling, fluid retention.

Common Immune Conditions: Rheumatoid Arthritis, Diabetes Type 1, Lupus, Fibromyalgia.

WHAT OTHER ORGANS CAN AN UNBALANCED GI AFFECT?

An unbalanced GI affects all body systems/cities in the United States of You since they all depend on the GI for nutrients! It is the "engine" of your car! The symptoms vary and include some of these below but this list is by no means exhaustive and there can be just one of these symptoms or a combination:

Brain city: including mental/emotional
Depression, irritability, brain fog/cloudy or slow thinking, memory lapses, lack of focus, anger, panic attacks, anxiety.

Ears, Eyes, Nose, Mouth, Throat
Long term postnasal dripping; headaches/migraines; vision problems; teeth/gingival problems; enlarged tongue; difficulty swallowing even without a nodule/growth; frequent ear, eye and or sinus infections.

Lung city/Respiratory System:
Frequent: colds, flus, pneumonia, bronchitis; difficulty breathing, shortness of breath.

Heart city/Cardiovascular System:
Palpitations/strong heart beats; too slow or too fast or irregular heartbeats; chest pain.

Endocrine System   Thyroid and Adrenal Gland county problems.

Kidney city/Urinary System
Peeing too often, difficulty peeing, incontinence/leaking.

Reproductive city/Gynecological System
Premenstrual syndrome, heavy bleeding, having no periods/cycles; low libido/sex drive, tumor/cyst formation like fibrocystic breast disease, ovarian/uterine cysts.

Musculoskeletal System:
Osteoporosis/Osteopenia (bone loss or weak bones); weak muscles; bone or muscle pain; cramps/muscle spasms; joint pain and or joint swelling.

General   Effortless weight gain or loss; excessive sleepiness/fatigue/lethargy; insomnia/poor sleep

Skin/Nails/Hair: Dry/rough skin; acne; rashes; psoriasis; eczema; fragile nails/break easily. Color changes in skin; thinning or excessive hair growth.

WHAT LAB TESTING IS COMMONLY DONE TO DETERMINE GI FUNCTION?
If you take your car to a mechanic for an engine problem, you expect him to look under the hood right? Well, to determine GI function we must look at all aspects of the GI-imaging such as endoscopies, colonoscopies, ultrasounds and X rays look for major problems, unfortunately if it is not an obvious problem these tests may come back as normal. That means we must now use very detailed testing, these are not typically done in the conventional medical system, so we refer to it as specialty testing. The three most common GI specialty tests are:

- **Complete Stool Analysis with Culture and Parasitology X 3-** *gives information on digestive system function-number of digestion bacteria, enzymes, parasites, inflammation and more.*
- **Heidelberg/Gastrogram Test-***measures production/levels of stomach acid*

- **Food Allergy Panel**-*analyses a BLOOD sample to see if your immune system/internal police are attacking 96 different types of common foods: meats, fish, dairy, nuts, fruits and veggies. Your immune system could react to new foods you have never tried before or even to foods you ate YEARS ago but have since stopped eating!*
- **Diet Diary*** *this is not a lab test but very useful to make food and symptom correlations*

WOW! NOW I SEE WHY ALL DISEASE AND HEALTH BEGINS HERE!

This is why I decided to specialize in this area because truly "you are what you eat" I love this region in the United States of You! It is VITAL to health! Fix your "Hole in the Middle"!

HOW CAN I HELP MY BODY RESTORE DIGESTION HEALTH?

By tidying up your tummy for total health naturally! You and or your friendly naturopathic doctor (me!) can look for the underlying cause(s) striving to remove them, if possible, while giving the body what it needs like vitamins and or minerals and getting back in tune with Nature's 9 Health Laws so that it can rebuild! **You can do this!**

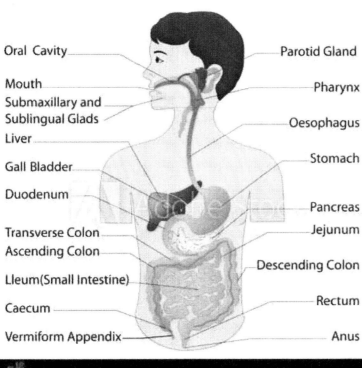

Oral Cavity

Mouth
Submaxillary and
Sublingual Glads
Liver

Gall Bladder

Duodenum

Transverse Colon
Ascending Colon

Lleum(Small Intestine)

Caecum

Vermiform Appendix

Parotid Gland

Pharynx

Oesophagus

Stomach

Pancreas
Jejunum

Descending Colon

Rectum

Anus

Biology   Digestive System

CHAPTER 5: A fun health story, so you can see how all the parts work together!

Now that you have learned so much about your body and its parts, I thought I would just give you a little story so that you can see how all of the parts work together. This story is an example of how your body will respond to an infection. So enjoy it!

Brain city/command center operator: *Prinnng! Prinnng!* Telephoning all sectors in the United States of You--- please send a status report.
Chest region: Heart and Lung city are all clear! *Thump! Thump! Breathe. Breathe.*
Abdomen region: Digestion cities are all clear! *Gurgle, Burp! Poop!*
Kidney and Bladder region: We are flowing smoothly! *Splash! Pee!* All clear!
Skin city: no cuts or bruises anywhere so we are all clear!

Now one day, the United States of You is opening a letter that a friend wrote to you, and after opening the letter, you accidentally get a paper cut on your hand. The evil Benny Bacteria is crawling around outside on your skin just waiting for the right moment to invade your country and as soon as he sees the paper cut/door open to the United States of You he sneaks inside!

Skin city operator to Brain city: *Prinng! Prinng!* Help! We are bleeding/semi-trucks are running off the road!

Brain city to Heart city: *Prinng!* We have a breach in sector 12—the hand! Please close down a few lanes on the highway/blood vessels in that region, so that more trucks do not run off the road! Also, make way for the platelets/glue road repair trucks to get to the area because there is bleeding! We must stop this right away!

Meanwhile, the dastardly Benny Bacteria gets onto Highway 75 North thinking to himself "Ha! Now, I am inside at last! And because I am an evil genius I will make my way north to Lung city where I can REALLY do some serious damage"...*moo hooo ha haaa ha!* (evil laughter)..."I have to be careful though because I do not want the police/immune system to catch me". Benny gets on Highway 75 north and makes his way to the lung. Benny is still undetected since Brain city was a little distracted with fixing the problem at Skin city. Once in Lung city, Benny Bacteria starts blowing up neighborhoods in Lung city...

Lung city to Brain city: *Prinng! Sniffle! Cough!* We think we might be getting sick...can you send over a police patrol car/immune cells please?

Brain city to chest lymph nodes/local police precinct: Please respond to a possible home invasion in sector 4-the Lung.

Chest lymph nodes to Brain city: copy that command center. Sending two officers to check it out. Over.

The two police cars/immune cells arrive at Lung city and discover the evil Benny Bacteria in Alveoli Neighborhood where he has taken a few innocent lung cells hostage.

Two Police officers to Benny: Give it up Benny! We have you surrounded! Put down your weapon!

Benny to Police: Forget it you dirty coppers! Moo hoo ha ha (more evil laughter). Meanwhile, Benny Bacteria finds an equally evil wife, Barbara Bacteria and they decide to make a lot of evil baby bacteria...since that is what bad bugs do...they get inside of you and then multiply so that they can increase their numbers to take over the United States of You! ☹

Two Police officers to Brain city: requesting backup in the Lung! Benny is putting up a fight! Please send back up on the double!

Lung city to Brain city: *Prinng!* Help! We are really under attack now!! *Cough! Cough!* We are drowning! *Achooo! Sneeze! Chest pain! Mucus! Phlegm! Gasp!* We cannot breathe well! The Benny Bacteria Family have completely invaded Lung city and we cannot get rid of them! *Gasp! Cough! Hiccup!*

Brain city to Heart city: *Prinng!* We have a MAJOR breach in sector 4—the Lung! Please speed up your beating! This is a level 10 orange alert! ***Danger! Danger!*** We must fight this infection fast!

Heart city to Brain city: copy that command! *Thump! Thump! Thump! Thump!* **Brain city command to Digestion city *911 Immune division*:** dispatch the SWAT/Special Weapons And Tactics police team to Lung city on the double! We have a serious infection! Also, initiate the fever protocol so that the police officers can drive twice as fast on the highways/blood vessels! We want them to drive 100 miles an hour! I repeat: initiate fever protocol immediately!

Digestion city 911 Immune division to Brain city: copy that command center! Dispatching SWAT bomb squad to Lung city as well as more police cars!

Then the SWAT van and the police cars get onto Highway 75 North and *flyyyyyy* up 75 North at 100 miles an hour to catch Benny! *WRRRR! SIRENS! FEVER! FEVER! WRRR! SIRENS! BLUE AND RED LIGHTS! FEVER!*

Brain city to _Digestion city Food Handlers_ division: shut down all digestion! Leave the meat, salad and whatever else United States of You ate for lunch on standby! We need all energy directed towards catching and killing Benny Bacteria and his family! Also slow down pooping!

Brain city to Kidney/Bladder Region: Slow down the water works! We do not have time for peeing right now! We need to catch Benny!

Kidney city to Brain city: Copy that command center! Niagara Falls has been temporarily shut down!

The SWAT team finally arrives at Lung city and immediately begins setting up their special bacteria bomb.

SWAT police to Benny Bacteria: last chance Benny! Surrender!

Benny to SWAT police: You will never take me alive! HA! *(even more evil laughter)*

Lung city cells: help us! Please! *Cough! Achoo! Cough! Sneeze! Runny nose!*

The SWAT team quickly finishes putting together their special bacteria bomb and rolls it close to Benny. Benny is so distracted by wreaking havoc that he does not realize a bomb is near him until it is too late...

Benny: Oh no!!! It is a bomb! *BAMB! BOOM! BOOM! Explosion!*

SWAT police to Brain city: Benny the Bacteria and his entire family have been blown up. A few innocent lung cells were also injured so please send ambulances and a repair crew to clean up Alveoli Neighborhood.

Brain city to Heart city: dispatch a repair crew to Lung city and an ambulance.
Heart city to Brain city: copy that command! *Thump! Thump! Thump!*

Lung city to Brain city: Lung city is cleaned up, and Benny's family remains have been packed up in the dump trucks and sent down to Digestion city! No more coughing, sneezing, chest pain or mucus! We cannot thank you and all of the other cities enough for saving us! Thank you!

Brain city to Lung city: You are welcome! All in a day's work!

Now that the infection is gone, all systems return to normal.

Brain city to Digestion city _Food Handlers Division_: resume digestion operations! Break down that salad! And send Benny's remains out to sea via the poop shoot!
Brain city to Digestion city _911 Immune Division_: please stop the fever protocol and send the SWAT team back to headquarters.
Brain city to Heart city: you can slow back down now to a regular beat rhythm. Reopen all highway lanes so our semi-trucks can begin delivering food and goods again!
Brain city to Kidneys: reopen the waterways!

Then the brain continues to monitor all events as if nothing ever happened...

Brain city command center operator: _Prinnng! Prinnng!_ Telephoning all sectors in the United States of You--- please update status report.
Chest region: Heart and Lung cities are all clear! _Thump! Thump! Breathe. Breathe._
Abdomen region: Digestion cities are all clear! _Gurgle, Burp! Poop!_
Kidney and Bladder region: We are flowing smoothly! _Splash! Pee!_ All clear!
Skin city: no cuts or bruises anywhere so we are all clear! Over!

Brain to all regions: Good job guys! Keep up the great work! ☺

CHAPTER 6: Can my body really heal itself of any illness?

Yes, your body can heal itself of anything and no, I am not making that up! As long as we are following the 6 main principles of naturopathic medicine:

1. **THE HEALING POWER OF NATURE**—the body can restore FULL health to itself!
2. **FIND THE CAUSE(s)**—Search for the underlying problem(s) of illness.
3. **TREAT THE WHOLE PERSON**-we are not just parts and organs, but mind, body and spirit.
4. **DO NO HARM**—generally avoid treatments that harm <u>any</u> part of the body!
5. **DOCTOR IS TEACHER**—learn about Nature's 9 Health Laws so you can heal your body!
6. **PREVENTION**—using Nature's 9 to avoid the development or worsening of illness!

In the conventional medical system (western medicine), remember that they usually do not hold to the healing power of nature principle, nor do they typically use any natural therapies. Therefore, under that system, the body usually cannot heal.

They do not often see people heal from a long-term illness and therefore will not tell you that you can heal! However, I, as well as many of my mentors who have been in practice 20, 30, 40 years or more have seen firsthand people restore FULL and total health to their bodies NO MATTER WHAT THE NAME OF THE DISEASE WAS OR HOW ADVANCED!

3 SITUATIONS IN WHICH A PERSON WILL NOT HEAL

There are usually only three reasons that a person will not heal *situation (1)* **The protocol is not strong enough for the illness**. Since no two naturopathic doctors will think exactly alike, you may have one doctor who will create an intensely powerful healing protocol and another doctor that may create a mediocre one compared to what is necessary for an intense illness. *Situation (2A) and (2B)* **the patient does not carry out a strong protocol intensely enough for what the illness requires because the patient is** *situation (2A)* simply too lazy to do a naturopathic protocol because they are used to just "taking a pill" and waiting for an effect to happen. Naturopathic medicine and getting back in tune with Nature's 9 Health Laws <u>requires effort</u> and for the patient to be <u>VERY proactive</u> about their health! Dr. Malcolm Johnson[32], Doctor of Oriental Medicine and owner of Godobe Health Services in Atlanta explains conventional medicine participation versus naturopathic medicine participation in a way I love. *Thanks for letting me borrow this Dr. Johnson* ☺.

Analogy: Pretend that you and I are inside of a building and I tell you, "hey let's go outside to your car. Then I pick you up, carry you outside of the building all the way to the parking lot, I open up your car door, place you inside your car and then close your car door. You would have very little to no effort/participation required right? That is the conventional medical system's participation level for the most part...just take a pill and wait to see what happens. The opposite is true of naturopathic medicine participation level. Again I would say to you "hey, let's go outside to your car" but instead in the Nat med model, I wait for you to stand up, we both walk out together to the parking lot (I do not carry you), you open up your own car door, get inside your car and close your door after you! See the difference?

Sometimes a second reason a patient is not able to participate intensely enough in a strong protocol is because **situation *(2B)*** they are currently too weak (physically or mentally) to do so and the patient does not have enough back up support from family or friends to help them to do the protocol until they can become strong enough to do it on their own. Finally **situation (3)** it is just that person's time to go. The power and timing of life and death does not reside within human hands...whether you believe it is God, Buddha, Allah, the universe, astrology, or whatever other higher power/entity that you may believe in, we know that we humans do not control life and death. Babies as well as old people die, sick or perfectly healthy people die. Therefore, if it is a person's time to go, then obviously that may be a reason why they will not heal. However, I always tell patients no matter how serious the illness is/how advanced in stages, I always say let us do this intense health plan with a passion!

Since usually neither I, nor you the patient, have received a letter/email/text message from the universe saying that you the patient is not going to heal, let us not just assume that it is your time to go! You have heard the saying that refers to an opera performance "it's not over until the fat lady sings" right? Well, I say let us give 100% effort, get back in tune with Nature's 9 and then we will see if the fat lady sings or not! In my experience, as well as that of my mentors who have been in practice much longer than I, the fat lady WILL NOT SING, but instead she just sits back down and watches you restore health to your body! **You can do this!**

CHAPTER 7: Oh no! I'm doomed if I don't decide to make a change today? Why?

TOP 10 KILLERS IN THE US in order: (1) Heart Diseases **(2)**Cancer **(3)**Long-term lower Lung diseases **(4)**Stroke **(5)**Unintentional injuries **(6)**Alzheimer's disease **(7)**Diabetes **(8)**Kidney disease **(9)**Influenza and pneumonia-more Lung diseases **(10)**Suicide .[1] The top two Heart Disease and Cancer kill over 50% of Americans! Heart disease alone kills more than 600,000 EVERY YEAR! Most of these killers are caused in great part by your lifestyle! Let us look at the first one: heart disease.

HIGH BLOOD PRESSURE

This is one of the most common heart diseases. I am sure that you know someone with high blood pressure, or maybe you have it yourself. Therefore, since this is such a common illness, people do not take it as seriously as they should because we hear about it all the time. **For example,** what is the most COMMON dangerous thing that we all do nearly EVERY SINGLE DAY? I will give you a minute to think about it...*nice elevator music is playing while you are thinking...* Did you answer get in the car and drive? Well if you did, you are right! Every time you get into your car, you are literally taking your life into your hands! Why? Because you are operating a very heavy object at high speeds, and you are sharing the road with sleepy, drunk, under medicated/OVER medicated, distracted drivers who are texting/talking on cellphones or fixing their hair/makeup! Even when YOU are following the rules, THEY may not be doing so and they can cause a serious accident!

But because it is so common for us to drive our cars, none of us are getting into the car, biting our nails and worrying will this trip be our last drive on earth or not! We are worrying about business meetings, bills, and school/tests and getting the kids to events on time and everything BUT driving! But just because it is very common for us to drive a car does not mean that it is any less dangerous! Same thing with high blood pressure, it is so common that people do not take it seriously. Having high blood pressure is the same as being hit with a hammer all over your body! It is just that you do not usually feel pain or get symptoms until it is at a very serious level!

Note: when you go to the doctor's office/hospital, what are the four things that are *always* checked by the assistants/nurse? **Temperature, breathing rate, heart rate and blood pressur**e. Do you know why we always check these four? Because if these are either too high/too low (temperature or blood pressure) or too fast/too slow (breathing or heart rate) then you could die in a matter of minutes to hours depending on the cause!

We call these four health markers **"vital signs"** because they have to stay in balance, as they are vital to you remaining in the land of the living! You see that one of those markers is blood pressure! *People are often more afraid of hearing the word "cancer" but we do not check for cancer markers at routine doctors' visits because cancer does not kill you fast. The average cancer takes years to kill* but high blood pressure is one of the most common reasons a person will have a heart attack or a stroke and either one of those can ABSOLUTELY KILL YOU IN 5 MINUTES OR LESS! You may not get any symptoms or warning signs that they are coming. We do not call high blood pressure the "silent killer" for nothing! If you have a heart attack or stroke, trust me it will be at the WORST possible time it could happen.

Now I know that you are thinking "Dr. Megan, there is NEVER a good time to have a stroke/heart attack!" That is true, but let me explain. What I mean is that you will not have a heart attack or stroke while you are at home lying in your bed. It will probably **happen under one of the** following **three** scenarios: *scenario 1* while you were carrying your baby and walking down the stairs, causing you to get dizzy and fall down the stairs with your baby in your arms. Or maybe *scenario 2* it could happen while you were driving and you pass out and your car goes into the lane next to you and you crash into a family with children killing 2 members of the family and paralyzing another member.

These are TRUE stories that have happened to people! These people have SO much guilt! They have either killed or injured and thus forever changed a few innocent people's lives because of a health problem that they knew about. Either they decided to ignore it completely — perhaps by not taking their medications and changing their lifestyle; or perhaps they always intended to start working on their health but never did. Often times, these individuals, and perhaps you too, did not realize what a serious health issue high blood pressure is. Even if you are taking medications but your blood pressure is STILL high, then that should be a sign to you that the problem is not under control and you have work to do! **Scenario 3a and 3b** are also bad. These involve what happens to you directly: **scenario 3a** obviously, you could have a heart attack or stroke and die. You would be gone and that would be the end of the story for you☹ . Just think of your poor family's shock over your death, also having to deal with the financial stress of burial and rearranging their lives without you! ☹ **Scenario 3b** is how the long-term effects of high blood pressure will slowly kill you over time. Maybe you have a stroke/heart attack and it does not kill you but you end up paralyzed or you cannot care for yourself as much anymore. **I do not know about you but I do not want to wear a diaper or have someone else wipe my bum for me!** *Sorry if that gave you a bad mental image.* ☺Or maybe you will not have a stroke or heart attack but Heart and Kidney cities begin to slowly stop working because of this constant "pounding pressure" they have been getting for months and years.

Now with two of your MAJOR cities working badly the entire United States of You is seriously weakened and you may have to be hospitalized or maybe one of your family members has to quit their job to try to stay at home and care for you.

You have added **three burdens** to your family: A *mental emotional burden* because they are sorry to see you suffer this way and want to help you. They may feel guilty if they cannot help you—especially if they have to put you in a care facility or if they cannot visit you in the hospital as often as they would like to; a *physical burden* if they are the ones caring for you because it takes ENERGY from them to care for you! Thirdly, but definitely just as important is the *financial burden* you have added onto them! Healthcare is ridiculously expensive and now they have to worry about your medical bills and the house bills too! *Therefore, if you do not act now, you are adding preventable long-term stress to your family members/friends and you are essentially STEALING THEIR HEALTH FROM THEM!* This may sound harsh, but I see this DAY in and DAY out and it is the truth*!*

Accident: You cross the street. A drunk driver hits you. You are completely paralyzed. Your family has to take care of you. You are not a TRUE burden in that case. **On the other hand, once you have the knowledge and the ability to make a change in your health and you do not change, that is when you may become a burden to your family.** Ok, I am tired of talking about blood pressure but I just had to do this because it is SO underappreciated and SO deadly. Let us talk about an illness that people are more afraid of cancer.

CANCER

It can be terrifying and very overwhelming to hear the word cancer if you or someone you know has been recently diagnosed! You may feel as if time has stopped and you are so afraid! Do not despair! Take a deep breath and calm yourself. **Most** cancers are **very** slow acting/growing. This section will help you understand what happens with cancer and with knowledge and understanding come power! You will hopefully feel less confused and fearful and have a clear picture of what has happened and even more importantly, how the body can respond to this injury!

Statistics

In the United States, more than 1,665,000 people are diagnosed with some type of cancer every year! The cost of cancer in 2009 was $216 billion! Cancer is the second cause of death in the United States. **Top three cancers** in the United States for **MEN (1)** Prostate **(2)** Lung **(3)** Colon/Large Intestine; **WOMEN (1)** Breast **(2)** Lung **(3)** Colon. Both prostate and breast cancer have numerous lifestyle factors associated with their development. Lung cancer is almost exclusively related to tobacco use/exposure and colon cancer is largely related to a bad diet, constipation/unhealthy bowels and lack of exercise.

Did you know that lifestyle and environmental factors may contribute to 90% of cancers?[2] Also, many experts agree that nearly 50% of ANY type of cancer develops in us because of these top 4 lifestyle factors that WE CAN DIRECTLY CONTROL such as tobacco, alcohol, diet, and obesity/inactivity![3] That is astounding!

What is cancer and how does it develop?

Cancer is an illness that develops from one of **your own cells/houses** when the body has lost the ability to control itself. A normal cell has **a life cycle** like a human in that, it is born a "baby" becomes a "teenager" and an "adult"-has its own "children" goes through "middle age" and then it grows old and dies. Genetics/DNA program most of the cells in our body to die when they get old...so they essentially "commit suicide" once they have fulfilled their "duty" to their country. However, a cancer cell turns "crazy"/mutates and decides it does not want to die and just continues to have children that also will never die. The backup system you have in place for cells that do not want to commit suicide after faithful service to their country is through your immune system/your internal defense: police/army/navy/air force in the United States of You. The immune system will recognize that Mr. Crazy Cell has become old and should have "retired"-eternally speaking-but since Mr. Crazy Cell was rebellious, your army cells/immune system will approach Mr. Crazy Cell and take him away where he will be "forcefully retired" or killed by your immune system.

The immune system controls all cells that become "crazy" because this can be happening at ANY given time and in any organ or part of our body. Crazy cells can develop in a healthy person, but especially in a person with ANY long-term illness because when you are sick over a long period you force your body to make new cells or "babies" **more often** than the body normally would because the body is trying to heal itself. Whenever the body is making new cells there is the possibility that a "crazy" cell can develop! However, if the immune system is ALSO not working well, then Mr. Crazy Cell's rebellion is too strong for the body, he begins to continue to multiply/make more crazy babies like himself, and the body does nothing to stop him because the body is too weak. Indeed, some of the new cancer cells DO die, but many more of them live since they multiply very quickly...like how rabbits can have 10 babies at once and be pregnant many times a year! Pretty soon the cancer cells/rabbits just start piling up on top of each other...some dead, some alive, all at different ages and sizes and steadily and rapidly multiplying!

Not considering the fast growing cancers like testicular (men) and pancreatic cancers, most cancers take at least 10-20 years before we can detect them with XRAY or some other imaging such as an MRI or CT scan. Remember that all cells in the body (whether normal cells or cancer cells) are **very** small and we

cannot see them until there are LITERALLY billions of them piled on top of each other and then they show up as a tumor/mass on imaging or you feel a lump.
Analogy: Cells are so small that it would be like trying to find one specific bunny rabbit in the ENTIRE UNITED STATES! It would be hard to find a bunny rabbit even just in your neighborhood or city, much less the entire country. However, if Mr. Bunny Rabbit found Mrs. Bunny Rabbit and they had billions of baby bunny rabbits (that never die and stay together in one place) then after a while there would be an area with a bunch of bunny rabbits. We could fly over the states in a helicopter and see 1 billion bunny rabbits in a pile easily from the helicopter. Understand?

What are the symptoms that cancer (crazy) cells may be developing?
Since most cancers grow slowly over 10-20 years, most people will not see any obvious or dramatic symptoms. However, these would be the signs to look out for when contemplating crazy cell development, which spells the word "caution"
- **C**hange in Bowel (pooping) or Bladder (peeing) habits
- **A** sore or bruise on skin that does not heal over weeks or months
- **U**nusual bleeding or discharge (like mucus or pus) from inside the body like in pee/poop or from the nose/eyes/ears/mouth/skin
- **T**hickening or lump/bump on or in the body (breast, arms/legs etc.)
- **I**ndigestion (constant) or difficulty swallowing
- **O**bvious and persistent change in your skin or in a wart or mole-- change in color, size, sensation-itching/burning/warmth
- **N**agging cough, hoarseness or persistently short of breath/difficulty breathing

What does benign versus malignant mean?
A crazy cell is **benign** if it **(1)** stays in the area of your body it was "born" into-like if it is a stomach cancer cell it stays there in the stomach and does not go to your liver or somewhere else in your body **(2)** does not change the type of cell it is—
Analogy: meaning if it was a circle cell it does not change into a rectangle cell
(3) does not actively destroy the location where it is. *Analogy: If you were trying to write, I come over, and I hold one or two of your fingers on your writing hand, I slow down or even stop the function you were trying to do which was to write but technically, I am not destroying your hand.* Now remember, the fact that it is growing and taking up space is *still damaging* the location where it is because it slows or stops function **(4)** if surgically removed it will not likely grow back **(5)** will have a typically "normal" size and shape for the area it came from. A **malignant cell** will do the EXACT opposite of all of the things above: it will change the type of cell it is, if surgically removed it may grow back, it may have all different sizes and shapes from its original beginnings and will actively destroy the area it is in.

42

Analogy: *you are writing, I come, I pull the pen out of your hand, and I begin stabbing your writing hand with the pen until your hand is practically useless!*

What is metastasis?
Analogy: *After I finish stabbing your hand, then I begin to move to other parts of your body and stab you anywhere that I can such as in the foot, leg, thigh, face etc.* That is what happens with crazy cells that are malignant, they will try to take their "we will never die" rebellion on a "road tour" all around the United States of You! They will travel most likely along your highways/blood vessels and your side streets/lymphatic vessels and go to other cities/organs in the United States of You if they can! ☹

How is diagnosing and monitoring of crazy cells done? What lab work or imaging is used?
The official way to diagnose any cancer is with a biopsy: using a needle to pierce and then pull out a piece of the organ or body part that we think might be cancerous and then looking at that little piece under a microscope. In some areas, it may be too dangerous to put a needle into it (such as the spleen and liver) because that area may have too much blood traveling through the organ or part and there is a high risk of bleeding with the procedure. Other times a biopsy is not done because it may not be an easy area to reach such as a tumor in the brain. Therefore, additionally, lab work and imaging is done- as well as using whatever information the doctor(s) have from a physical exam. A common physical exam is feeling a lump on the breast (women) or feeling the size of the prostate (men). I know you men hate this "finger" exam. Believe me, it is not fun for us doctors either☹. Sometimes multiple organs may be affected. To monitor progression/speeding up or regression/slowing down of the illness, usually the same exams are used. These common tests are done usually in combination:

- **Basic Blood work:** looking at red blood and white blood cells, all basic organs functioning. Some crazy cells can increase or decrease the body's production of normal substances like hormones and enzymes, which will be reflected in the blood work.
- **Specialty Blood work:** some crazy cells release substances that are not usually in the body that we can measure with lab work known as tumor markers. They can be organ specific...like one marker is released only if a person has breast cancer versus substances made only if a person has prostate cancer.
- **X-rays/Radiographs:** shows picture changes in body region densities/thickness

- **CT Scan:** uses high powered x-ray to show a horizontal cut across an organ or body region
- **Endoscopy:** shows a direct view of a hollow body cavity/passageway (like throat/stomach/colon)
- **Ultrasound:** uses high frequency waves to show density differences, especially solid versus fluid.
- **Magnetic Resonance Imaging (MRI):** uses magnetic fields and radio frequencies to show a cross section/cut across view of the body organs and structures.
- **Biopsy:** removing an actual piece of the organ or part and looking at it under the microscope. We see how the cell has changed from what it should have been. Biopsies can be done using a fine needle, pulling out fluid, a skin punch, endoscopy or with a surgical cut of the area.

How are crazy cells classified?

Most crazy cells are classified as either benign or malignant. Additionally, malignant cells are classified based on the amount of development they have (grading)—again this is like a crazy cell that was born and got to be "middle age" and then died. While another cell may die as a baby. The staging of cancer refers to how extensive or how much the disease has progressed. Some cancers have their own unique grading and staging systems but in general grading and staging will look at three factors:

- **Tumor:** the location(s) and size of the origin or first tumor/primary tumor
- **Nodes:** lymph node (part of your lymphatic system/side streets) involvement or if any tumors are there.
- **Metastasis:** spread to any other organ or part of the body besides the site of origin (primary site)

How are crazy cells treated in conventional medicine?

In conventional medicine, there are five main forms of treatment:

- **Surgery**—removing the entire organ or part of an organ or area where crazy cells are found
- **Radiation**-using high energy radiation to damage crazy cells (includes ionizing radiation and particle beam radiation)
- **Chemotherapy**-uses medications to slow down/stop cell: growth, development, reproduction or metastasis.
- **Hormonal Therapy**-some cancers are strengthened by hormone levels so decreasing the amount of hormones available to the crazy cells will weaken them

- **Immunotherapy/biotherapy**—combines biological agents with chemotherapy or radiation for desired effects. Includes bone marrow transplantation, monoclonal antibodies and colony stimulating factors

How does naturopathic medicine approach crazy cells?

Since naturopathic medicine is a field that is not <u>completely</u> controlled by protocols, as is conventional medicine, you will find that naturopathic doctors' views on how people with crazy cells should be approached can be quite varied depending on the doctor. **Note:** 7 or 8 out of 10 conventional medical doctors may give the same answer for how to work with a person who has cancer, while asking naturopathic doctors how to work with that same person, you may get only 2 out of 10 to give you the same answer!

- Some naturopathic doctors may prefer to use **100% conventional medicine** only (drugs and surgery) while only supporting the body with natural therapies in between conventional treatments.
- Other naturopathic doctors may be more comfortable using **50% conventional treatments and 50% natural therapies** or some other mixed percentage.
- Other **naturopathic physicians would prefer a 100%** only naturopathic protocol.

My own view is that one should look for the underlying cause(s) of why your body allowed crazy cells to develop. Try to remove those causes if possible, at the same time doing heavy duty cleansing of the body to get rid of trash. Give the body what it lacks (vitamins, minerals etc.) and get it back in tune with Nature's 9 Laws of Health. In this way, the body can try to restore health to itself as it already can do, like when you get a cut on your hand. In using 100% natural elements that in general do not harm the body but ONLY help the body, then we are helping the body in the best and most optimal way.

How do I determine which way(s) to pursue?

Obviously the ultimate choice is YOURS, the patient, as to which approach you would like to pursue, and your physician(s) should support your decision whether they are conventional or naturopathic doctors. However you need to actively research and ask for information from conventional and or naturopathic doctors to help you make your decision. Understand that the philosophies in their respective fields will dictate the advice or information they pass along to you about your illness.

Conventional Medicine General Philosophy

- There are some illnesses that are incurable and once you have it you will always have it and therefore all that can be done is to palliate/make you more comfortable.
- If a part/organ of the body is no longer functioning then you remove it—if possible, replace it with another organ or machinery.
- The main therapies are drugs, surgery, physical therapy and radiation
- There are protocols to follow once a diagnosis is made, with no emphasis on treating the person as an individual.
- Conventional medical schools do not train or study natural methods nor teach body restoration—therefore they may not be willing OR even able (by the governing medical body) to direct you to try something outside of their protocols. Doctors can get into legal trouble for recommending a treatment outside of protocols and or their specialty area. Therefore, they will STRONGLY discourage you from straying away from the normal conventional treatments.

One must understand that the typical treatments used in conventional medicine (drugs, surgery and radiation) are in general not specific enough to hurt only the cancer cells. Therefore, they damage and kill healthy cells as well not just in the area where there is cancer, but also they weaken the entire body. This is why most people undergoing cancer treatment get so sick and have numerous side effects. *Analogy: It is like if you had a deep cut on your right hand and so you just put a bandage on the hand to cover the wound. Every couple of days you have to change the bandage on the right hand, but when you change the bandage on the right hand, you have to smash the left hand with a hammer.* To my mind, this is what happens when treatments are used that work to get rid of a symptom/problem in one area of the body, but at the same time are damaging another area of the body. The medications, radiation and surgery may be working on reducing tumor size etc. but they are also damaging other cities in the United States of You- particularly the digestion and immune systems.

Do not misunderstand me! Conventional treatments can be VERY useful in some situations, perhaps in smaller doses, more spread out and if included with mostly natural medicine could be more effective for certain cancers/individuals! It just depends on the individual and the type and degree of cancer. In general, most cancer treatments are invasive and very harmful to most people in most situations.

Naturopathic Medicine General Philosophies

- The body can restore health to itself, one must help it do so, especially if the body has become overwhelmed and lost the ability.
- We should try to rehabilitate/heal a damaged part/organ and not simply remove it or replace it.
- If we use natural therapies that work with the body and help it to heal, without damaging another part of the body, that is more effective.

As long as you understand all risks and benefits of using either one and or both systems, you can then make an informed decision about how to proceed. **Whatever method (s) you choose you must be 100% at peace with your decision, your family and friends may or may not support you, but in the end, it is your body and your decision no matter which way(s) you choose. You are also free to change your decision too. Just remember that if you are picking a more destructive or permanent option (like removing a body part) you cannot UNDO that decision later.** You should also be at ease with being able to openly share with your physician(s) your health desires, fears and goals and you should feel that your physician has heard and supports you and has informed you about all positive or negative aspects of any procedure or plan. Always try to get the most information from all sources (physician, internet, books, other individuals) regarding any operations, procedures that are to be done or any medications to be taken including short-term and long-term side effects, risks versus benefit.

NOTE: Keep in mind that even if you do pursue a conventional treatment that all you need is for ONE malignant cell/rabbit to survive chemotherapy, surgery or radiation and the whole process begins again.

I have beaten cancer twice or multiple times! That is good right?
No! I have heard people say how they have beaten cancer multiple times but that is NOT a good thing to have cancer "leave" and return! Remember, to develop cancer in the first place, you have to have a failure in two systems: **(1)** the cell itself –failed to "commit suicide" at the proper time **(2)** the immune system failed to kill the crazy cell that decided not to die. *Analogy: A foreign country invades the United States. Imagine, the enemy country's soldiers just coming out of submarines and or parachuting down into our neighborhoods, or even walking into our country from a landlocked neighbor and our military did nothing to stop it! Or maybe it is not even a foreign country, but a few of our own citizens who decide to turn crazy and overthrow the government! Again, the local police do not take action!*

This is supposed to be one of the strongest countries with the best military and technology right? So if we were invaded or had a rebellion **even once**, we would ask ourselves what went wrong? Does our air force and navy need better radar systems for planes and boats approaching our coasts? Do we need better training for the army and police on the ground? What do we need to change so that this does not happen again? We would definitely make those changes after **one** such incident, and *especially* if it happened twice or more because the more times we allow our country to be overtaken the more chances we have that one day the invaders/rebellion will be successful! ☹ The United States asked itself those same questions after the horrible terrorist attacks on September 11, 2001 and you can see the changes that the government has made in our country in how we fly and many other situations just based on that ONE event. So now do you see why "beating cancer" many times is not a statement to make proudly? Instead, you should ask yourself what went wrong, and immediately get back in tune with Nature's 9! **You can do this!**

Is there a certain way to eat if I have cancer?
Yes! This illness is a little different from others (just like Diabetes) and requires a more specific nutrition plan. Nutrition is vital to creating health! Digestion involves breaking down foods from large sizes to microscopic sizes and pulling out the vitamins and minerals we need from them. We want to use foods that are easy for the body to digest so that the energy we save can go towards rebuilding the immune and entire system**! In addition, digestion requires more energy if you eat a meal versus if you drink vitamins/minerals in a drink**. This is typically why emphasis is placed more on fluids than meals; FOR EXAMPLE: you can easily drink 50 carrots but you could not easily eat 50 carrots! A drink will allow you to gain the nutrition of 50 carrots without having to chew so much or waste energy in breaking down 50 carrots!

What are the main nutrition concepts?
During "boot camp" the first 2-4 months minimum after diagnosis main points: **(1)** We want to **avoid "feeding" cancer/crazy cells** and they love SUGAR! Especially from processed forms (cookies, cake, soda) but they will also use carbohydrates (bread, rice, cereal, pasta, potatoes, and fruit) because these foods are high sources of sugar. Why avoid sugar? It gives them energy! **(2) Avoid animal products** (anything that had a mother at some point is an animal product). Why avoid animal products? They take more energy to digest/break apart and they tend to have more bacteria or other stuff we do not want in them. We do not want to waste energy on breaking down food. We want to use food high in nutrition but use the least energy possible. We definitely do not want to take in more toxins/trash either **(3) Avoid processed** or prepackaged foods. Why? Because the packaging process makes them very low in vitamins, minerals, and we NEED EVERY vitamin and mineral to rebuild your body! **(4)** We **need protein** to rebuild a system so average 30 grams to 50 grams a day is good.

(5) Food preparation: no microwaving food to cook it, no deep-frying, no baking food. Why not? High heat destroys vitamins and minerals! Again, we need to get the maximum benefit from the food! So again here is the list:

Eliminate:

- *PROCESSED FOODS*: anything precooked or premade from a box, bag, bottle, can or wrapper! EAT ONLY FRESH FOODS FROM MOTHER EARTH! Organic if possible, but if not just wash food very well. Home cooked.
- **NO SUGAR/HONEY/CANDY**
- **NO POTATOES, RICE, BREAD, PASTA, CEREAL.** Eat an especially low starchy/carbohydrate diet.
- **NO FRUIT**--first month. After that avoid or limit more starchy/sugary fruits like banana, dried fruits (raisins, apricots etc.), pears and focus more on berries-blue, black and raspberry. Only one serving of fruit daily.
- **NO MEAT OR FISH**—if too low energy then maybe just a serving or two a week
- **NO DAIRY**—anything from a cow (milk, cheese, butter, yoghurt, creams)
- **NO EGGS**
- **NO SALAD DRESSINGS**—can make your own dressing from olive oil, salt, Braggs Aminos are fine. Can add lemon and herbs to season!
- **NO EATING OUT:** no junk food, fried foods, fast food OR eating mixed foods that others prepared (IE a casserole your family made and you do not know the ingredients) unless you get salad without dressing on it.
- **BEVERAGES:** Water is your main drink now. NO CAFFEINATED DRINKS (coffee, sweet tea, energy drinks); NO SODA; NO JUICES—especially fruit juices! Exception: veggie juice you made yourself with juicer, but still use veggie juices sparingly and dilute with water.

So what in the world does that leave me to eat?!?

Beans, green veggies, nuts for that first month at least and then you add in a little fruit in month two etc. However, again, this is all very individual and you have to base what you are doing on how you feel. Very important to work with an integrative health professional(s) if one is available.

NOTE: I NEVER ask anyone to do something that I have not tried myself and although it takes planning this is very doable! You can eat really well and feel great!

Analogy: Do you see why I call the first 2-4 months "boot camp"? Boot camp in the military is a time when the body, mind and spirit undergo many difficult changes in a short period. After the first few weeks in military boot camp, the body and mind become more used to all the changes and it gets easier to keep going! Likewise, these first few months are VERY difficult but important in you gaining ground in helping your body begin to rebuild! As you make new habits, your body will begin to respond and it will get easier!

Some meal ideas for crazy cells (but these are healthy meals for anyone)
During "boot camp" it may be best not to have certain items-like animal products-but again the actual plan depends on the individual. Most of these foods have studies showing that they have some crazy cell fighting properties! Here are a few ideas:

BREAKFAST
- **Cereal:** a handful or two of a mixed nuts with ½ cup of blueberries and/or raspberries and almond or soy milk
- **2 Boiled eggs** with a small apple and half an avocado
- **Mushroom and spinach with ground flaxseed**, steamed tomatoes and an apple
- **2 scrambled eggs** with onions, broccoli and red pepper.
- **Smoothie:** 1 cup of almonds, 1 large avocado, 1 cup of berries, 1 cup of soy or almond milk-blend in the blender

LUNCH/DINNER
- **Bean salad** (white beans, green beans, red beans) with tomato and red onions
- **Tomato and basil soup** with kidney beans
- **Romaine lettuce salad** with broccoli, olives, tomato and avocado and steamed tofu
- **Mushroom soup:** Reishi, Shitake, Maitake, Bella, White (the first three are the best) add in meat, beans or tofu with steamed broccoli/carrots.
- **Slightly steamed/cooked whole tomatoes** with garlic and mackerel.
- **Stir-fried purple cabbage** with carrots, mushroom and 2 cups sliced almonds.
- **Avocado, red onion, black bean** and spinach salad.

SNACKS
- **Raw broccoli heads**/carrot or celery sticks with hummus-chickpea or garbanzo bean-spread
- **Mixed raw nuts** with a ½ cup of raisins
- **Fruits** serving sizes: berries-1 cup, pineapple-1 cup, apple-1 small one, raisins-1/4 cup—max fruit allowance per day is one serving.
- **Artichoke and cumin dip** with raw veggies-steam artichoke and then blend in blender with salt pepper and cumin. Then dip in raw veggies.

Use plenty of crazy cell fighters such as garlic and onions; healthy herbs and spices such as rosemary/thyme/basil, turmeric and oregano.

Cancer summary

Breathe! You have time! If we focus on getting ALL citizens of the country to be on the lookout for cancer cells/rabbits and to call emergency 911 if they see one, and we also rebuild our police/army/navy/air force then the ENTIRE system will become strong and take back the "country"! *Analogy: like when the US was looking for Bin Laden after the Sept 11 terrorist attacks...remember how everyone knew what he looked like because they showed his face on all TV channels, on the internet, all over the country and world! Even small children could identify him, and of course, especially our military so that eventually EVERYONE was primed to catch him. It was only a matter of time before he was caught because EVERYONE was on the lookout for him!*

That is what I propose to help the body to do. Instead of only focusing on cutting out or drugging crazy cells, wherever they may be, let us instead focus on why your two systems of protection failed. Let us help your body rebuild those systems and the entire United States of You by using Nature's 9 Health Laws and using mainly only helpful natural elements so that the body can restore health to itself! **You can do this!**

STROKE

This happens when there are not enough semi-trucks/red blood cells getting to the different areas in the brain. There are two types **(1)** traffic accident/blood clots or **(2)** semi-trucks running off the road/bleeding. Many things can cause strokes but one of the most common reasons is high blood pressure. There can be temporary or permanent damage in the brain after a stroke, it just depends on how long that area went without blood. The after effects will depend on what area did not get blood, so if it is in the back of the head where your vision is controlled you can become blind. If it is on the side of your head where movement is controlled, your whole body or certain limbs may not move as well, or not move at all.

Risk factors for having a stroke:

- **High Blood Pressure** or any other heart disease: Atrial Fibrillation, Congestive Heart Failure etc.
- **Diabetes**
- Cigarette smoking
- **Alcoholism**
- High Cholesterol/other fats in blood
- **Having already had a stroke** or a heart attack
- Using certain birth control pills
- **Obesity/too much extra body weight**
- Having a prosthetic/fake heart valve
- A **lifestyle** with low physical activity/exercise
- A bad diet allowing hard plaques to form in your blood vessels/heart roads. We call this Atherosclerosis. Excess sugar helps this happen ☹.
- **Family history**
- Age: older than 55 years old
- **Race:** more common in African Americans/Blacks
- Gender: more common in men

Of course the more of the risk factors you have the worse it is☹. But remember, you can change most of these risk factors☺.

Signs and Symptoms of a Heart event

Here are the most common signs and symptoms that you or someone you know may be having or about to have a stroke or heart attack in the next few hours, days or weeks. The symptoms may come on suddenly and intensely or be new but persist slowly over time. Symptoms usually occur only on one side such as having a weak left arm but could also be on both sides. The symptoms could last only for a few seconds or for minutes or hours:

Stroke:

- Weakness in the hand, arm or leg; difficulty in reaching for objects
- You **cannot move** a body part well or at all: hand, leg, toe, finger, arm, foot
- Drooping of your eyelids or lips
- **Difficulty** speaking or finding words
- A VERY strong headache
- **Blacking out** or feeling like you lost consciousness for a second or two
- Changes in your vision: loss of vision, blurry vision or double vision
- **Changes in sensation**: you cannot feel or tell the difference between hot or cold items, soft or hard or you feel numbness in hands/feet/arms/legs

- Mental confusion: you do not know the day, month or time

Heart attack:
- Chest pain—dull, sharp or pressure like pain
- Men: **Jaw or arm pain** is very common
- Women: can more often have back pain instead of arm pain or abdominal pain/upset stomach
- **Sweating** a lot without exercising
- Difficulty breathing/shortness of breath
- **Indigestion or heart burn**
- Sense of impending doom or **strong fear**: this just means your body will let you know that something is VERY wrong and that you had better go to the hospital. Many people will get this feeling but not always.

Another serious heart event: A blood clot in the leg
A blood clot/traffic jam in the leg can form from sitting too long without getting up from time to time. A few examples **(1)** a long flight minimum 3 hours or more **(2)** sitting all day long in the car or at work **(3)** a recent surgery, which restricts your movement, can lead to a traffic jam in the leg. The traffic jam/clot will cause a dull or achy pain in usually only one leg. You may also feel numbness in the leg, feet or toes. This blood clot is bad in the leg but what really makes it serious is when the clot breaks free from the leg area and travels up to Lung city where the roads are much narrower and then it causes a full highway shutdown in Lung city! The symptoms will be chest pain, shortness of breath or difficulty breathing.

THIS IS A LIFE THREATENING EMERGENCY SO GO TO THE HOSPITAL!

Lung city is the top of all organs...remember after approximately three minutes without air you will faint! If you do not receive treatment then soon after that you will die☹. Avoid sitting all day long and if you must sit then try to get up and walk and stretch every two hours to keep blood moving.

A HEALTHY person should do this minimum. **If you have any illness** like Diabetes, High Blood Pressure/another heart disease or an Autoimmune disease **then you have EVEN MORE RISK of having a blood clot/traffic jam!** Therefore, you need to keep your legs moving and drink plenty of water to keep your blood/semi-trucks from sticking together! Additionally you should avoid sugary foods and drinks when you know you have to sit for a long time. **Remember this phrase "sticky and greasy on the outside is sticky and greasy on the inside".** For example, honey is sticky right? It makes your fingers stick together on the outside of your body. Honey/excess sugar will also make your red blood cells/semi-trucks stick together on the inside too! Most people do not abuse honey but they do abuse sugar! Fried foods are greasy and too much grease makes things stick together on the inside also!

If you get these heart event symptoms or see the signs in someone else, get them checked out! Remember that sometimes when we do lab work or imaging it is too early to see the problem so even if at the hospital they tell you everything is fine, but you know that you still feel badly do not be afraid to insist!

ANOTHER HORRIBLE KILLER: DIABETES

This illness is usually a SLOW MEAN killer but sometimes it can cause conditions that can kill you FAST too. It is SO SNEAKY! It can make people lose all kinds of body parts/functions and leave a person completely messed up. That is why I hate it! TONS of people have diabetes, it has become very common, and so people do not take it seriously. I want to spend quite a bit of time explaining it so that it can help you or people you know with it. It can be very overwhelming to understand diabetes and blood sugar control if you were recently diagnosed or even if you were diagnosed years ago! Perhaps you do not have diabetes yet but are pre-diabetic. This section will help you understand what is going on with diabetes and blood sugar control! You do not have to read it in one sitting-although you can if you want to! However, you can read a few pages at a time, always reviewing the other pages you read before moving on to new pages, and then little by little you will see how you begin to understand the concepts, remembering them and better yet USING them!

What are the current statistics of diabetes?
Unfortunately, this illness is extremely prevalent in our society as well as in the world. The Centers for Disease Control (CDC) states:

- 26 million diabetic patients in the US.
- 79 million pre-diabetics
- Demographics
  - 11% of people 20 years or older
  - 27% of people 65 years or older
- 1 in 3 born will be diabetic
- 1 in 2 Hispanics/Pacific Islanders
- 350 million diabetics worldwide.

What is the cost of Diabetes in the United States?
- 2007: $174 billion
    - $116 billion in excess medical expenses: hospital in-patient care, diabetes medications or supplies, treating complications, physician office visits.
    - $58 reduced national productivity
- Average diabetic patient costs a year: $6,649 attributed to diabetes.
    - $1 out of $5 health care dollars in US is spent caring for someone with diagnosed diabetes.
    - $1 out of $10 health care dollars is attributed to diabetes

What types of Diabetes exist?
There are two main categories of Diabetes:
(1) Diabetes Mellitus--includes Type 1 Diabetes/Juvenile/Autoimmune Diabetes, Type 2 Diabetes, Latent Autoimmune Diabetes of the Adult, and Gestational or pregnancy induced Diabetes.
(2) Diabetes Insipidus.
- **Diabetes Type 1** occurs when your body's immune system/your internal police force gets confused and attacks the pancreas-the organ that would help produce the Insulin hormone needed to help keep blood sugar/glucose balanced. This usually is diagnosed very early in life (childhood) and people must take insulin. 5-10% of people with diabetes have this form.
- **Latent Autoimmune Diabetes of the Adult** occurs usually around 35-55 years old where the immune system attacks the pancreas but just later on. Patients are often misdiagnosed with Diabetes Type 2.
- **Gestational/Pregnancy Induced Diabetes** occurs only with pregnancy and can be due to hormonal changes related to pregnancy. Typically Diabetes will go away after birth, but developing gestational diabetes could be a sign that a person could be at risk to develop Type 2 Diabetes later on.
- **Diabetes Insipidus** is a very rare form that occurs when either the body does not produce enough anti-diuretic/anti-pee hormone, or if the kidneys do not respond to the hormone when it arrives to the kidneys. The two main symptoms are excessive thirst and excessive peeing. Very rare.
- **Diabetes Type 2** is when the body does not produce enough of the hormone Insulin to control blood sugar, OR the body produces enough insulin but the body's cells do not respond to the insulin. This is THE MOST COMMON FORM of Diabetes—90-95% of people who have Diabetes have this form so it will be the focus of this section.

A few analogies to help you understand!

- **Analogy Number 1:** Remember your body as the United States of You. You have these main areas-- the north, south, east and west. Think of each of your body's organs as cities so you have Heart city, Brain city, Lung city, Pancreas city, Liver city etc. Each city is composed of groups of neighborhoods, and the smallest unit would be a cell or ONE house. Each cell/house in every city is responsible for producing items that its region and overall "United States of You" needs. We then transport all internally produced supplies (vitamins/nutrients) to your organs/cities in semi-trucks/red blood cells that travel along your highways/circulation system and the side roads/lymphatic system. The Gastrointestinal system/Digestion city is more like a region in the US of You (like the south) because it is comprised of 3 parts/counties the Mouth, Esophagus, Gall Bladder and 5 organs/cities the Stomach, Small Intestine, Large Intestines/Colon, Liver and Pancreas. Digestion city receives all <u>outside</u> supplies—vitamins and minerals from your food and beverages--and then distributes them to the rest of your cities/organs using the semi-trucks/red blood cells via your interstate system/ circulatory system (heart pumping). See Digestion city chapter 4 if you need to review. Another important area in the United States of You will be Adrenal Glands county.

- **Analogy Number 2:** We will refer to blood sugar/Glucose as "teenagers" and Insulin as the "chaperones" for teenagers.

- **Analogy Number 3:** Later when we discuss how the body responds to certain blood sugar levels we will also refer to Insulin as a "salesman" and Glucose as "cookbooks".

- **Analogy Number 4:** Carbohydrates are fast or "rabbit energy", while protein is slow or "turtle energy".

What is blood sugar, where does it come from, why do we need it?
Blood sugar/glucose is the main quick energy source for the body. The brain gets about 90% of its energy from using blood sugar/glucose. All other organs in the body constantly use it too and so do muscles for movement. We get most of our blood sugar from food especially carbohydrates and proteins but from beverages that have sugar in them like soda, teas, coffee, and juices. However, because blood sugar is so important, the body can make it too. The liver is the organ that makes it and stores it for later use. When we need to make blood sugar Adrenal Glands county releases a hormone called Cortisol that travels to Liver city to let it know we need more blood sugar on our highways. At the same time Pancreas city makes another hormone called Glucagon, which also goes to Liver city to increase release

of stored blood sugar. The blood sugar then gets onto the highway/blood circulation (accompanied by Insulin/chaperones) and travels to different organs/cities. The blood sugar goes into the individual cells/houses that will use blood sugar for their day-to-day activities. The body must maintain a minimum amount of blood sugar. We need more during the day because we are more active, and less at night because we are sleeping, but there still must be a basic minimum of blood sugar available at all times in our blood highways and in our cells/houses because it is our main energy source.

What is the main problem if someone has Diabetes type 2?
Essentially your body has a problem with keeping your blood sugar/glucose balanced. Remember our teenager and chaperone analogy #2? We need a certain amount of glucose/teenagers out on the highways/blood circulation at any given time. We do not ever want TOO MANY unsupervised teenagers out at one time because they tend to get into trouble—drinking, driving too fast, taking drugs etc. Often when many teenagers get together without adult supervision, they do things they would not do if they were alone. We also cannot have TOO FEW teenagers out either because we need them to work and make energy for us in ALL regions of the United States of You. If your body is working properly, we have the right amount of teenagers out and we make sure they stay out of trouble by making the Insulin/chaperones accompany them. Our Insulin/chaperones are coming from Pancreas city. However, if we have a problem making Insulin/chaperones OR if the cells/houses do not allow the glucose/teenagers to come inside the houses then we may find ourselves with too many unsupervised teenagers/glucose driving around on our highways/blood circulation and causing serious problems.

How does someone develop type 2 Diabetes and who is more at risk?
Many factors make you more likely to develop it:

- **Age**-risk increases with age beginning at about 30 years old and older
- **Weight**-having a body mass index (BMI) of 25 or higher, if Asian a BMI 23 or higher. Abdominal/belly fat can especially increase blood sugars
- **Blood Pressure**-more than 140/90 or higher. High top or bottom number
- **Cholesterol and lipid levels in blood**-Low HDL--this is the "good cholesterol". Low is less than 50;Triglycerides 250mg/dL or higher
- **Family History**-having a parent, brother or sister with Diabetes
- **Ethnicity**-being Black/African American, Hispanic or Native American puts you at greatest risk, than does being Asian or a Pacific Islander. Whites/Caucasians have the lowest risk
- **Diabetes in pregnancy**

- You were **born having a high or low birth weight**—you weighed more than 9 or less than 5.5 pounds
- **Inactivity**-exercise fewer than three times a week

Other countries where Diabetes is projected to rapidly increase in the next 30 years: will increase by 50% in England, 72% in Australia and New Zealand, and 184% in Mexico!

What are the symptoms if blood sugar is too high or too low?
Blood sugar/glucose can at times be too high or too low. With type 2 Diabetes it is often too high. Many people have NO symptoms at all until the blood sugar has been high for a while.

- **High Blood Sugar (Hyperglycemia):** fatigue, frequent peeing-especially during the night, extreme thirst, constantly feeling hungry, effortless weight gain or weight loss, headache, numbness and tingling in arms or legs, vision problems.
- **Low Blood Sugar (Hypoglycemia):** hunger, irritable/anxious, dizziness, fruity breath, unsteady walking, cold sweating, confusion, pale face, palpitations/strong heart beats, numbness or tingling of tongue, lips or fingers, trembling, slurred speech, decreased memory, warm/hot feelings, abnormal behavior.

  At blood sugar levels less than 50-55 mg/dl this is potentially LIFE THREATENING! A person can begin to have seizures, lose consciousness and even go into a coma. SEEK MEDICAL ATTENTION. This occurs most often in those with Type 1 Diabetes but can also occur with people with Type 2 Diabetes. It usually happens if someone **(1)** takes too much insulin and or **(2)** does not eat or eats too late after taking insulin **(3)** is taking medications or illicit drugs that stops Liver city from making blood sugar or **(4)** increases high/intense exercise without first lowering insulin.

IT IS MUCH MORE DANGEROUS TO HAVE TOO LOW BLOOD SUGAR THAN TOO HIGH BLOOD SUGAR.

What are the long-term health risks of uncontrolled or high blood sugar?
Glucose/blood sugar is sticky so it causes "stickiness" of semi-trucks/red blood cells, so they run into each other and get stuck causing "accidents and traffic jams" on your highways/blood circulation. A traffic jam in Heart city is a **HEART ATTACK**, a traffic jam in Brain city is a **STROKE**. Glucose can also cause traffic problems (but not actual traffic jams) in Kidney or Heart cities leading to **KIDNEY FAILURE** and **HEART FAILURE** respectively, which will lead to water building up all around your body (edema) and also to **HIGH BLOOD PRESSURE**. Traffic jams often occur in the eyes which is why Diabetes Type 2 is the LEADING CAUSE of **BLINDNESS**. Stickiness

of red blood cells in limbs, but especially in the feet and legs often prevents a person from feeling when they get an injury-like a cut or wounds in the foot. This is because the nerves that would let the brain know about the injury are also "sticky" and cannot send messages back up to the brain very well. Also, Semi-trucks/red blood cells in these areas are in traffic jams, so then this prevents the cut/wound from getting vitamins it needs to heal. Therefore, it does not heal well or at all, and if this goes unnoticed by you or someone else, an un-healed wound over a long period can lead to foot or leg **AMPUTATIONS**. These are the main long-term effects but many more are also possible because the ENTIRE BODY/UNITED STATES OF YOU suffers.

What are the guidelines and lab work used to diagnose type 2 Diabetes?
We can measure **(1)** fasting glucose–you have had no food or beverage except water for minimum 8 hours **(2)** random glucose—measured at any time-regardless of whether you have eaten or not
 (3) Hemoglobin A1c measures your average blood sugar over the past three months.
- **Fasting glucose**—normal is between 70-100 mg/dl. Fasting more than 126mg/dl is Diabetes
- **Random glucose**—after eating your blood sugar should be between 120-140mg/dl. Random glucose more than 200mg/dl is Diabetes.
- **Hemoglobin A1c**—normal is 4.8-5.6 mg/dl. More than 6.4 mg/dl is Diabetes
- **Pre Diabetes** is a fasting blood sugar between 100-125mg/dl *OR* random blood sugar between 100-199mg/dl, or a Hemoglobin A1c 5.7-6.4 mg/dl (this means that your average blood sugar is 130-145mg/dl)

Other parameters that could be measured for diagnosis are C-Peptide which is a part of Insulin production and fasting Insulin.

What are the main daily factors that affect blood sugar?
- **Food and Drink**—THIS IS THE MAJOR PLAYER in blood sugar regulation! **(1)** what you eat **(2)** how much you eat and **(3)** when you eat it are ALL very important in keeping balance!
- **Water/hydration**--not drinking enough water/being dehydrated will make a "sticky" situation even stickier!
- **Exercise**--can affect blood sugar, depends on the intensity--walking is less intense, jogging, swimming, bicycling are way more intense and can greatly affect.

- **Stress**-emotional or physical can lead to an increase of blood sugar because of the stress hormone Cortisol made in Adrenal Glands county that travels to Liver city. Remember one of Cortisol's jobs is to increase blood sugar.
- **Sleep**-poor sleep can also lead to increase in Cortisol and raise blood sugar. That is because low sleep is a stress on the body.
- **Dawn phenomena**-blood sugar is normally higher in the morning even in people that do not have Diabetes. Because you have not eaten all night, in the early morning Adrenal Glands county will send the stress hormone Cortisol to Liver city to tell it to release blood sugar so that we can have energy to start the day. So for a person who has diabetes, their morning blood sugar will be extra high!

What food types can affect blood sugar?
- **Carbohydrates/carbs**--this is the MAIN group that we need to restrict/limit! Remember analogy #4? This category of foods is ALREADY blood sugar--it does not need to be broken down into sugar by Digestion City so it is fast or "rabbit energy". As soon as you eat carbs, you are releasing TONS of "teenagers" (analogy #2) onto your highways/blood circulation without supervision! This will raise your blood glucose very high VERY FAST! *Carbs are Rice, Bread, Potatoes--or anything made from potatoes like potato chips or French fries, Pasta, Fruit, Vegetables, Cereals (hot or cold), Pancakes, Milk (cow and goat), Crackers, Juices, Candy, table sugar, honey and artificial sweeteners.*
- **Protein**—this is slow or "turtle energy" because proteins are like a chain necklace with many links in it that is tangled at the bottom of a bag. Digestion city workers first must untangle the necklace and then remove each of the individual chain links. This takes a few hours to do, which is why breaking down protein does not raise your blood sugar quickly. However, since protein will EVENTUALLY break down into blood sugar-just more slowly-you also have to watch how much you eat of it. *Proteins are Red Meats (beef, bison), Poultry (chicken, turkey), Fish, Beans/lentils, Nuts, Tofu/Soy products, Egg Whites.*
- **Fats**—these foods will NEVER break down into blood sugar in the body so you can eat these in unlimited amounts. Only oils are 100% fat. Choose healthy oils such as olive, coconut and almond oils. However, two foods that are 60-80% fats are avocado and coconut. Avocado has higher fat than coconut. Although be careful because they also have carbs!

BOOK ALERT: Woo Hoo! One fourth of the way through the book! ☺

What are special circumstances that also affect blood sugar?

These situations could also greatly influence blood sugars either increasing or decreasing blood sugar:

- Medications
- Infections anywhere: pneumonia/in lungs, flu, urinary tract/pee roads, dental, stomach
- Trauma
- Surgery
- Alcohol

What are the ways that blood sugar is controlled?

Diet and then weight control are the most important ways to regulate since NO amount of prescribed medication will compensate for OVEREATING sugars! Carrying a lot of extra weight (especially on the stomach) increases blood sugars! However, medications are also used in the following ways:

- **Oral/taken by mouth medications only-**Metformin is very common
- **Injectable Insulin only-**must inject with a needle or pen or can wear a pump
- **Oral medications and Injectable Insulin together**
- **New INHALABLE Insulin!**—*No more needles! The U.S. Food and Drug Administration just approved it in 2014! Dr. Sam Shum and his team at MannKind Corporation created the device.*[62] *Learn more about it on their website!*
- **Many herbs can help** ONLY once diet and weight are being controlled

What is the ideal diet for blood sugar control?

Just as with Cancer, Diabetes has a more specific eating plan than does any other illness. Since Carbohydrates (rabbit energy) is the MAIN food category raising blood sugar, you will need to restrict these. **You CANNOT simply eat what you want and add more herbs, oral blood sugar medications or injectable insulin!** Proteins (turtle energy) will also have to be limited. *Fats do not need to be limited because they do not ever break down into blood sugar.* Foods in packages will state the amount of grams or ounces of a food so that you can measure them. BEFORE MAKING ANY MAJOR CHANGES TO DIET OR MEDICATIONS, YOU MUST CONSULT WITH YOUR PHYSICIAN(s)! You will have to read packaging labels to see how many grams or ounces of each of these categories are in each SERVING SIZE of the food. The ideal ratio to maintain blood sugars in great ranges would be the following:

- **Carbohydrates---30-45 g daily**—eat the highest amount at lunch or dinner and the lowest carbs at breakfast. Remember the morning glucose is higher already due to the dawn phenomenon, which is when Cortisol hormone from Adrenal Glands county travels to Liver city to have it release more sugar so we can get our day started since blood sugar was lower during the night while we were sleeping.

EXAMPLE: If you were eating 30 grams of carbs a day then breakfast might be 6 grams of carbs and then lunch 12 grams of carbs and dinner 12 grams of carbs.

- **Proteins**—eat protein with each meal to help you feel full and slow down the speed of blood sugar from the carbs you eat. The amount of protein at each meal depends on body weight. **The formula in general is 0.8-1.5 g of protein/kilograms of body weight/per day.**

EXAMPLE: MATH ALERT!! ☹
If we have a 200-pound person, how many grams of protein should they eat in a day? First we must know that <u>ounces/oz are the standard measurement used on packaging for meat, fish, and poultry</u> and that 1 oz of meat is 6 grams of protein that will turn into glucose.

First, we must convert pounds to kilograms before we can use our formula so we know that 1 pound/Lb. is 2.2 Kilograms (kg). **Secondly,** divide 200 lbs. by 2.2 kilograms, which equals 90.9 kilograms. **Third,** using the formula, we multiply 90.9 kg by 0.8 g of protein and that will equal 72.7 or approximately 73g of protein daily. To calculate how many ounces of protein a day, you need to divide 73 g of protein by 6 grams, which equals 12 ounces of protein. So based on what the package/menu says you could eat in a day either 73 grams of protein or 12 ounces of protein. Then we would evenly space out the protein amongst the meals.

Remember you can eat healthy oils unrestricted since they never turn to blood sugar/glucose.

What tools do I use to record and monitor blood sugar?
It is of VITAL importance to DAILY and REGULARLY check your blood sugar levels. There are many tools that can be used, how many of them you must use will depend on if you are taking oral medications only or also injectable Insulin. Mainly, there are supplies for monitoring glucose, using Insulin, and for correcting blood sugar imbalances. Your general doctor and or endocrinologist must prescribe some of these tools to help you with controlling blood sugar issues.

- **Glucometer**—instrument that measures blood sugar by testing a drop of blood
- **Glucometer Strips**—holds the drop of blood that will be placed into the glucometer
- **Glucometer Lancets**—the instrument that pricks your finger to get the drop of blood
- **Insulin Syringes/Needles**---used to inject insulin into certain areas of the body
- **Insulin Pen**—you can also use this to inject Insulin. Looks cooler than using a syringe. ☺ It is still a needle though. ☹
- **Glucagon Pen**—used in emergencies when blood sugar is too low. *Glucagon hormone tells the liver to release and to make blood sugar.*
- **Other low blood sugar products**-glucose tablets and gels—taken by mouth when sugar is dangerously low
- **Glucograph**—document that shows what your blood sugars were at different times of the day—fasting, after breakfast or dinner etc. Take care to write down the times!
- **Diet Diary**—this document is where you DAILY write down **(1)** EVERYTHING that enters your mouth: ALL food, beverages, gum etc. **(2)** their exact QUANTITIES for example: Dinner was 2 ounces of grilled chicken with 1 cup of broccoli **(3)** the TIMES you ate them. Additionally, you note how food was prepared: grilled versus fried and all sauces and ingredients the food contained.

Using the diet diary and glucograph together allows us to see where problems in blood sugar are happening. If your blood sugar is ever too high or too low at a particular meal or time then to investigate you need to look at the meal just BEFORE the imbalance happened to find the answer(s).

EXAMPLE 1: blood sugar is <u>too high at 7pm dinner</u> then you would want to look at what happened around *lunchtime*. Perhaps you ate a snack between lunch and dinner. Maybe you ate too many carbohydrates (rabbit energy) at lunch. Or perhaps you forgot to take medication at lunch?

EXAMPLE 2: blood sugar is <u>too low at 5am</u> and you wake up sweating and shaky with your heart beating fast. Look back at *dinner the night before*. Maybe you did not eat enough food at dinner. Perhaps you took too much medicine at dinner. Or maybe you exercised right after dinner and used up some of your blood sugar?

How often do I have to check my blood sugar/glucose?

Daily and regularly! Four times a day is optimal especially if you were just diagnosed or your sugars are not controlled well. Check **(1)** fasting--first thing in the morning or after 8 hours without any food or beverage except water. **(2)** after breakfast, lunch and dinner. However, often insurance will only pay for a certain number of strips so you may only be able to test once or twice a day. Taking the fasting morning sugar is essential as is measuring sugar at one other time in the day after a meal. You can speak with your doctor about writing a prescription for more strips.

I am on Insulin. What are the different types of Insulin and how do they work?

Most Insulin you must take orally/by mouth or inject with a needle. Insulin is like a chaperone for blood sugar. Remember analogy #2? Back in the old days teenagers could not go out on a date alone, they had to go with a friend, brother or sister to make sure that the teens did not get into trouble. Insulin is the chaperone that takes the blood sugar into your cells/houses. We use Insulin based on three factors (1) **Onset**--how fast the Insulin starts to work (2) **Peak**--time that Insulin is having its highest effect (3) **Duration**--how long the Insulin effect lasts. Generally speaking, you use Insulins close to meal times, and or at bedtime and to make corrections if blood sugar is too high. There are four categories of Insulin that are most commonly used: **(1)** Rapid **(2)** Short/Regular **(3)** Intermediate **(4)** Long acting Insulin.

- **(1) Rapid Insulin** --(Novolog/Aspart; Humalog/Lispro; Apidra/Glulisine)— Onset 15-20 min, Peak 30 min-2.5 hours, Duration 3-5 hours. *Used mainly at meal times and to make quick too high sugar corrections.*
- **(2) Short/Regular Insulin**—(Humulin regular/Novolin regular)—Onset 30-45 minutes, Peak 2-3 hours, Duration 4-6 hours. *Used mainly at meal times.*
- **(3) Intermediate Insulin**—(NPH)--Onset 2-4 hours, Peak 4-10 hours, Duration 10-16 hours. *Used mainly as a basal dose meaning it helps keep minimum glucose required by your body steady at all times whether day or night.*
- **(4) Long Acting Insulin**—(Lantus; Detemir)—Onset 2-4 hours, No Peak, Duration 11-24 hours. *Used mainly at bedtime only (basal dosing), or dosed perhaps twice a day at 12 hour intervals. Helps keep minimum glucose required by your body steady at all times whether day or night*

How fast does Insulin work? Which is worse taking too much or too little Insulin?

Oral blood sugar medications like Metformin, also escort sugar back home but MUCH more slowly than Insulin since the medication first has to go through Digestion city--which takes 1-3 hours. On the other hand, since Insulin is injected directly onto your blood highways it does not have to go through the digestive system and its effects are almost immediate. ***Analogy:*** *Oral medications gently tap the glucose/teenagers on their shoulders and saying* **"ok kids, time to go home now".** **Oral medications wait** *until the teens stand up and let the teens slowly walk to the car and then drive home. On the contrary,* **Insulin** *says to the teens* **"WE ARE LEAVING NOW!" It grabs the teens by their arms and drags them** *to the car, pushes them inside and speeds off to the house and then throws the teens inside the front door!*

Therefore, Insulin works so quickly that if you take TOO MUCH Insulin you can lower your blood sugar so fast that it is dangerously-life threateningly low! Below 50-55 mg/dl, if you are awake you can faint and then enter into a coma. Or if you were asleep, you can enter directly into a coma! Usually this crisis happens when people take Insulin right before a meal, and then forget to eat or do not eat enough food for the amount of Insulin they took. Sometimes people take Insulin at bedtime and take too high a dose. Then they often enter into crisis in the middle of the night. **Therefore, remember this rule: IT IS BETTER TO HAVE TOO HIGH BLOOD SUGAR THAN TOO LOW BLOOD SUGAR!** If you do not remember if you took Insulin or not at a meal or before bedtime, do not take any! Wait until the next meal or scheduled dose. Also, always eat right after you inject Insulin. Do not allow work, family or other things to distract you. Some patients take long acting Insulin once a day at night; others may need to take it twice a day at 12-hour intervals. If you are on Insulin, you **must** work very closely with your physician to get the dosing correct. Remember the dosing will also vary based on daily lifestyle factors and changes so this is a ***constant*** work in progress until you can help your body heal itself!

What is Insulin resistance?
Now we will use analogy #3. *Now Insulin is a salesman and glucose is a cookbook. Imagine on a Saturday or Sunday morning you have a salesman who knocks on your door offering to sell you a cookbook. You buy one about Asian cuisine. A few hours later, he knocks again to sell you a cookbook and you buy one on American cuisine. He continues to come by every few hours and you continue to buy cookbooks until you have every major type of cuisine as well as specialty cookbooks on subjects like desserts only, or kids' foods etc. He comes again the next day and wants to sell a cookbook, but now you tell him you have enough cookbooks. He leaves, but then returns hours later to sell more cookbooks. Now you are angry and you do not even open the door anymore when he knocks! However, since he is very annoying and persistent he just keeps on coming and knocking!* This is Insulin resistance! When you over eat carbohydrates and thus have too much blood sugar, we have to increase the amount of Insulin to cover all of this extra sugar.

Your body either increases making Insulin, or if you are taking Insulin, then the amount or dose has to be increased. The Insulin/cookbook salesman then escorts the sugar/cookbooks into cells/houses where the cells use the sugar/glucose for energy. However, after a while, the cells decide they do not want to take in any more sugar/cookbooks and then they will ignore the Insulin/cookbook salesman "knocking"! At this point, even increasing oral blood sugar medications or even increasing Insulin may not help the cells to take in blood sugar! This is a HUGE problem because then blood sugar can start building up outside of cells on your "streets/highways" and making very sticky situations/traffic jams!

If you have a "belly" or abdominal fat, then this is especially a problem that will happen! Why? Because belly fat sends a lot of salesmen to Liver city. The liver gets tired of "cookbooks" and no longer lets blood sugar in. However, we need blood sugar inside of our cells/houses constantly for energy to run the house. Since inside the Liver cells we are using and running out of glucose, at one point we have NO teenagers in the house to do chores like take out the trash, wash dishes or clean! In reality, the inside of our cells have no energy and are starving! This situation makes Liver city decide to make and put out blood sugar onto our highways. The liver cannot make sugar to use directly inside its own cells though. The liver has to accept sugar <u>from outside</u> of the cells/house. But since sugar is already high outside on the streets, when Insulin comes knocking on Liver city doors (or any other organ/city door) the cells do not open the door! Do you understand the vicious circle?

What resources exist for Diabetes?
Your doctor should be your #1 resource. However, many books and websites are useful. Remember that websites can disappear but one can always find books.

BOOKS

- <u>Diabetic Eye Disease</u> by A. Paul Chous, MD, OD: Fairwood Press

- <u>Diabetes Burnout</u> by William Polonsky: ADA

- <u>The Diabetes Athlete</u> by Colberg: Human Kinetics.

- <u>Dr. Bernstein's Diabetes Solution</u> by Dr. Richard Bernstein.

- <u>Type I Diabetes</u> by Ragnar Hanas, MD, PhD.

- <u>The Diabetes Travel Guide</u> 2nd Edition by Davida Kruger: ADA

- <u>Pumping Insulin</u> and <u>Using Insulin</u> both books by John Walsh, PA, CDE

- <u>Understanding Diabetes</u>, by Peter H. Chase

- Managing Preexisting Diabetes and Pregnancy, ADA, Kitzmiller, MD, Jovanovic, MD, etal.

- Start Pumping: A Practical Approach to the Insulin Pump, by Howard Wolpert, ADA

- Insulin Pump Therapy Demystified: An Essential Guide for Everyone Pumping Insulin by Gabrielle Kaplan-Mayer.

- Think Like A Pancreas: A Practical Guide to Managing Diabetes With Insulin, by Gary Scheiner, MS, CDE

WEBSITES

- http://www.diabetesincontrol.com: Dr. Bernstein's weekly newsletter

- www.childrenwithdiabetes.com: Comprehensive weekly newsletter for patients/physicians of Type 1 Diabetes

- www.behavioraldiabetes.org: California institutes focuses on the mental/emotional/behavioral aspects of having diabetes.

- http://www.barbaradaviscenter.org/: One of the leading clinics in the country who treat pediatric patients with Type 1 Diabetes.

- http://www.joslin.org/CME_Index_2231.asp: One of the leading clinics in the country treating diabetes.

- http://www.diabetesnet.com: Comprehensive site run by John Walsh, MD

- http://www.fda.gov/Diabetes/

- www.healthesolutions.com (I REALLY RECOMMEND THIS ONE!)

- www.fatsecret.com Gives the amount of calories of protein, fats and carbs of common foods.

Diabetes Summary

I hope this has helped you to feel a little more informed about how the body controls blood sugar and about Diabetes. You must work closely with a wise physician to regulate blood sugar, particularly if you are on Insulin. It is a hard process when you start learning-especially at the beginning because everything is new and it feels overwhelming! Take it slowly and do not get overwhelmed! Study this information until you have all concepts memorized! Remember that it takes time and energy to understand these processes. However, you will learn and you will daily make decisions that allow your body to begin restoring health to itself!

Thank you to Dr. Mona Morstein[61] for the nutrition and diabetes literature insights!

The problem with developing any long-term illness, no matter the name
We are often too lazy about our health! We blame genetics, everything, and everyone else. Instead of re-taking control of our health, we resort to drastic and dangerous methods—such as harmful medications and surgeries--to correct the issues--methods that generally only cause more damage and do not address the underlying problem—which is that we are out of tune with Nature's 9! We can cut, burn, radiate and drug away symptoms and the problem may temporarily _SEEM_ to go away, but later on IT WILL RETURN IN THE SAME ORGAN/PLACE or SOME WHERE NEW in the body but when it returns, it will return with a vengeance—a bigger and even meaner illness/disease than before! ☹

Wait Dr. Megan, you are yelling at me, but I did not even know about Nat 9!
Ok, sorry to be yelling at you if you did not know about these.☹ In addition, it is true that the environment/things outside of our control also act against us, and we do not always bring health problems onto ourselves...although we do contribute to our poor health MUCH more than we think! Anyway, if you did not know about Nat's 9 then ignore that I yelled at you, and move down to the next paragraph. But if you **did** know about Nat 9, just take the yelling understanding that it is meant out of concern and now move on to the next paragraph. ☺

TWO HEALTH MODELS: CONVENTIONAL and NATUROPATHIC
We touched on this earlier but I thought this would be a good place to explain further the strengths and weaknesses of the two systems.

Conventional Medical System	Naturopathic/Alternative Medicine System
Fast and Furious philosophy	Slow and Precise philosophy
Best for life threatening/trauma	Best for long-term illness (Diabetes etc.)
Best for reconstructive surgery	Best for short-term illness (cold, flu)
Think of it as the **"hammer"**	Think of it as the **"screwdriver"**

Originally, the **conventional system** was designed to handle emergencies. Therefore, the philosophy is that actions must be used which are immediate and powerful. This system is **EXCELLENT** at what it was originally **intended** to do! If you have been in a serious car accident and your lower leg was cut off they can reattach it! If you have a gunshot wound(s) they can find the bullet(s) remove them and stop the bleeding! If you were born without half of your face and you cannot eat because of it, they can construct a new face for you! THEY ARE FANTASTIC AT THIS! This is their strength.☺ The treatments are fast and furious (meaning aggressive) therefore in my analogy they will be the "hammer".

Unfortunately, in the 1800's and early 1900's people began to use the conventional system for NON-emergencies. Today, more than 60% of visits to the conventional medical system are for long-term illnesses. Since the system's philosophy is fast and furious (hammer), its structure does not work well for a person who is coming in with an illness that requires many questions to be asked and enough time to investigate the medical problem thoroughly (screwdriver).

You need to understand the strengths and weaknesses of each model so that you know when to use each system! WE NEED THEM BOTH!

THE FIVE MAIN ISSUES WITH THE CONVENTIONAL MEDICAL SYSTEM
(1) Emphasis on **specialization**/the specialists do not talk to each other
(2) No individualization-doctor makes diagnosis→ everyone gets the same treatment
(3) Treatments work against nature/body→leads to side effects
(4) Polypharmacy-using many different drugs→drug interactions create symptoms
(5) Doctors do **not** have **enough time** to spend with patients→leads to misdiagnosis

DISCLAIMER: I am speaking about two different healthcare models conventional and naturopathic. I AM NOT speaking against any individuals in the model such as doctors, nurses, or technicians. In the same manner that one may not agree with the concept of warfare, but not be against the soldiers.☺

 # 1 Emphasis on specialization/specialists do not talk to each other
The body is so complex that specialties developed in medicine so that a doctor can learn one specific organ/area very well. Trying to keep on top of all of the medical information for the entire body is very difficult. Over time, more and more doctors became specialists after general medical school. We do have doctors that continue to look at the entire body called general practitioners (GPs) or primary care practitioners (PCPs) or even family medicine doctors. Naturopathic doctors also train this way. However, there is more prestige and more money in specializing in a specific organ/area. That is one of the reasons that we have a shortage of general doctors in this country currently. Hence, you the patient may have to wait weeks or months before you can get an appointment with one. Now look at these areas and the doctors that treat them:

- **Brain problem**? →Neurologist
- Hormones out of balance? →Endocrinologist
- **Ear, Eyes, Nose or Throat issue**? →ENT/Otolaryngologist
- Heart problem? →Cardiologist
- **Lung problem**? →Pulmonologist
- Digestion troubles? →Gastroenterologist

- Have cancer? → Oncologist
- **Kidneys** do not work? →Nephrologist
- Prostate problems? (men) →Urologist
- **Joints swollen/painful**? →Rheumatologist
- Menstrual cycle or baby making problems? →Gynecologist/Urologist (men)
- **Muscle and bone problems**? →Orthopedic specialist
- Skin look like a newborn lizard? Spotted and greasy? →Dermatologist

Wow! That is many "ologists"! The problem with this is that each specialist is only looking at one area of your body. The conventional medical system does not allow the doctor to cross over into another area of your body because that is not their area of expertise. For example if you are visiting your heart doctor/cardiologist for a heart problem and the heart doctor suspects that your kidney markers-items the kidneys make or control-are bad, the heart doctor cannot just begin treating you with kidney specific medications. The doctor must refer you to a kidney doctor/nephrologist or else they could get into legal trouble. Your heart doctor will prescribe heart medications and the kidney doctor will prescribe kidney medications. Neither one of the doctors will speak to the other doctor about your case though. They do not have time. Depending on your current health picture, you can easily end up with 5 or more doctors!

 # 2 No Individualization: doctor makes diagnosis and all receive same treatment
The problem with this is that everyone receives the same treatment if people have the same diagnosis. Even though they have the same name disease, often the cause(s) of the disease are different and therefore the treatment should be different. ***Analogy:*** *let us say that we have two cars. Each car has a flat tire. The first car's tire is flat because there is a big nail in the tire. The second car's tire is flat because the tire valve cap keeps falling off while driving and the air leaks out slowly. The mechanic looks at both cars and sees that both cars have flat tires (the same diagnosis) and so he decides to refill both tires with air.*

Is this the best approach? To put air into both tires? Not really. Yes, both the tires do need air. However, the cause of the flat tire is different for each car. To fix the problem with the first car, the mechanic must remove the nail from the tire, patch the nail hole and then refill the tire with air. The second car tire needs to be refilled with air AND THEN have a tire valve cap put onto it. Unfortunately, in conventional medicine if two people walk into the door with same long-term disease (such as high blood pressure) the system treats both people with the same high blood pressure medication even though the cause(s) of their disease is different. The first person's blood pressure may be high because of bad food choices and the second person's blood pressure may be high because of high stress situations that make their stress hormone Cortisol increase their blood pressure. The treatment for the first person should be a nutrition change and the second person should look for ways to reduce or handle the stressful situations. Make sense?

3 Treatments work against nature/the body and cause side effects

Most pharmaceutical drugs stop one specific symptom or problem. They are made to work very quickly and powerfully (hammer). You see that the symptom is gone and therefore you think that you are better. That is not always the case. In fact most of the time the drug has only "hidden" the symptom so that now you do not feel it or see it anymore. The health problem causing the symptom is still there. Most drugs are powerful and overwhelm the body and in doing so, they will stop the body from trying to heal itself because the drug is so much stronger.

Note: The pharmaceutical companies must make drug doses much higher than what you actually need so that Liver city does not break apart the entire drug before it enters your blood/highways. We call this the **first pass effect**.

Analogy: Imagine that you are walking with a very small child or a dog. You pass a football field on your right where you can see a bunch of big, strong football players practicing. Suddenly, the child/dog runs away from you and will soon run into a busy street where there are many cars and trucks driving by. You panic! You call the child/dog to return to you but they do not listen to you.

You are about to run after the child/dog but then someone grabs your right arm and stops you! You turn around and it is a football player! You try to shake him off because you must get to the child/dog before it reaches the dangerous busy street! But the football player is too strong for you to shake off. You begin pulling him along. Then ANOTHER football player grabs your left arm! Now you are very scared because the child/dog is almost in the street! "Let go of me!" you scream at them both. But they do not listen to you. Now you are moving VERY slowly dragging two big football players on each arm but you are still trying to reach the child/dog before they get hit by a car! The child/dog is about to step into the street!!! You are really, really scared now! You are pulling the two players with all of your strength and then suddenly you fall to the ground! Why? A third football player tackled you from behind! You now have THREE big football players holding you and they are too strong for you to move anymore. All you can do now is move your head, yell, cry, and watch the child/dog go into the dangerous street. ☹

In this analogy, the child/dog is the symptom(s); you represent the body's desire to fix or correct a problem and the football players are conventional medications. We have spoken about this a little before. **Pain, fever or ANY other symptom is the body sending you signals that something is wrong and that the body has**

already begun to try to correct the problem. However, we do not like those signals and instead of helping the body we turn off those signals with medications that are not doing ANYTHING to help the situation--allow the child/dog to get into the street--and are instead making the problem worse by creating side effects or harming another area of the body.

4 Polypharmacy: using many different medications that create symptoms

Poly is a prefix that means "many" and pharmacy just means pharmaceutical or prescribed/over the counter medications/drugs. One medication can cause side effects on its own. If you add a second medication, not only can that second medication cause its own side effects, but the second medication can also begin to interact with first medication! Either the second drug will help the first drug work better or the second drug will make the first drug work worse or even stop the first drug from working at all. Additionally, sometimes the drugs will cause the same symptoms as the original disease and then it is very difficult to tell the difference between if it is the drug causing a symptom or if it is the disease causing the symptom!

Story: Once, I had a patient that came for stomach pain. They had already seen another doctor before who had prescribed a medication. They took the medication and their stomach pain got worse. The problem was that one of the side effects of the medication was ALSO stomach pain! I could not tell if they had stomach pain because the disease was getting worse or if it was a side effect from the medication. Can you tell? By the way, this is not an isolated case. Some antidepressants can cause depression...the very thing they were supposed to prevent! Other medicines also act this way. The symptoms that these drugs create can be in the same organ/city as the original problem/disease area or in a completely different organ/city or area. Very often, the symptoms they create are in a different organ/city.

5 Doctors do not have time to spend with patients. Leads to misdiagnosis.

Doctors would like to spend more time with you but they cannot because the system structure does not allow it. Why not? First, we must have some background knowledge. Medicine is vital to life. If something goes wrong in your body, we must find it and treat it or else you could die either quickly or slowly. The health insurance agencies (HMO and PPO) were created to help this problem by allowing you the patient to pay a small fee to receive the care that you need so that your life is not in danger. The health insurance agency helps doctors find patients to fill their private offices by putting a list of doctors on their plans. Then you the patient looks at the list of doctors in your area and pick the one(s) you need.

The health insurance company only requires you the patient to contribute a small fee (co-pay) towards your doctor's visit and then the insurance company pays the rest of the cost of the visit. Otherwise, your doctor's visit would cost hundreds of dollars...the same high price you pay when you go to see another highly educated and trained person such as an attorney. Again, because medicine can be life or death and legal matters usually are not, in this country we created the insurance system and a credit/debt system to help people have access to medical care at a more affordable rate. In other poorer countries if you cannot afford to pay to see the doctor (and no one can help you pay) then you just die☹.

Because the health insurance company is making it easier for doctors to get patients to fill their offices, by paying some of the cost of the visit, the health insurance company may impose some "rules" on the doctors. Meaning the health insurance company does not want a doctor to take too long in seeing patients. For example, if a patient comes in for a bleeding nose, the insurance company may say to the doctor you should be able to figure out what is wrong with this patient in 15 minutes or less. Now, the doctor has to follow these time constraints to some degree. If they go over the allotted time then the insurance company may decide not to pay the rest of the cost of the visit. Sometimes a bleeding nose may not have a simple cause though! Many insurance codes exist for all of the different symptoms.

Let us say that the co-pay is only $20 but the true cost of the visit is $300 because the doctor has to use supplies to look into your bloody nose etc. Remember that the insurance company does not pay the doctor the amount of money for the rest of the visit right away. The insurance company pays the doctor the rest of the money many weeks later--as long as there is no problem with the insurance paper work--so the doctor only earns the money you pay them that day!

Therefore, for that reason, doctors in private practice must often double and triple book appointments every day because each patient is only paying $20-$50 dollars. This is often why you experience long wait times at the doctor's office because the doctor may make three appointments for 8 o'clock in the morning and if ALL three of you arrive on time then automatically you have to wait. But if you all cancel then the doctor made no money.

If the doctor took a little too long on the visit and or perhaps the person who does the insurance billing and coding in the doctor's office did not use the proper insurance codes, the insurance company may decide not to pay the doctor the rest of the visit cost.

So that poor doctor only made $20 when he should have made at least $300! The doctor can try to argue with the insurance company but that usually takes weeks or months.

Now think about how much you pay for your own bills: rent, car, water and electricity bills. Do you have the amount in your head? Remember that a doctor in private practice has all of those bills twice! Why? Because they must pay those bills for their personal life AND for the practice. If you were having a house party and charging people to come to your house party, how many people would you have to invite in one day to cover YOUR monthly bills if each person was paying $20? The doctor has to come up with twice that amount!

Obviously then, the doctor has to see MANY patients in one day to be able to pay their bills. Since the doctor only has a few hours in each workday, they must spend less time with each patient. The average doctor visit is 10-20 minutes or less.

Because the doctor does not have enough time to spend with you--not because they do not want to but because the system is built that way--then they may not arrive at the right diagnosis (misdiagnosis) or perhaps they just make a general diagnosis that is not specific enough. However, you expect them to prescribe a medication for your symptom or problem and the medical system has protocols/rules for them to follow about how to treat certain symptoms or problems. They cannot change the system's established rules/protocols very much or else they get into trouble. Therefore, they see you for 10 minutes and prescribe a medication and then they move on to the next person. Remember, the doctors would LOVE more time with you. They simply cannot because of how the system is structured.

Saying: I have heard it said that the government (Uncle Sam) cannot make you do anything...but that instead it can make you very sorry that you DID NOT do something! The same is true for doctors and professionals working under the medical system. They have rules to follow, just as a soldier does at war. The doctors or soldiers may not like or agree with what they are doing but while they are working under that system, they must follow the rules or else they will be very sorry that they did not!

Note: Since most conventional medical doctors do not train in natural therapies, they do not know how they work and they cannot recommend them to you because they would not know how to manage your care with a product(s) with which they are unfamiliar. In addition, even if they WERE familiar with natural therapies--some doctors are and use them at home for themselves--doctors can face expensive fines, have their license taken away and or even go to jail for breaking protocols!

To become a doctor in the United States a person must complete 4-5 years of university, then 4 years of general medical school, and then if they decide to specialize there could be anywhere from 3-8 years more training depending on the specialty the doctor picks. The longest training specialty is surgery...for obvious reasons! Doing the math that **is minimum** 8 to 9 years of higher education to become a doctor! The average cost of general medical school *alone* is $200,000 dollars! Unlike some other forms of debt, the loan system does not forgive education debt after a period. Debt collectors chase doctors for that medical school loan money forever! Therefore, that doctor is **not** going to risk having spent minimum eight years of blood, sweat, and tears and not being able to practice their profession and possibly even going to jail on YOU! They will give you the standard medication and keep on moving.

It is hard to be a doctor: By the way, this is also a reason why there are actually high suicide rates among conventional medical doctors. There is NOTHING healthy about studying medicine! The 4 years of general medical school is very hard. However, the residency (training period after medical school) is the most intense. Little sleep, high stress: working with patients who do not feel well and therefore can often be very mean, the doctors supervising the less experienced doctor may ALSO be mean and you are doing all this with the pressure of knowing that if you make a mistake you can really hurt or even kill a person! This high stress lifestyle lasts for YEARS! Drug use is also a problem in medical training because depending on what stage of training they are in, they must work 60-80 hours a week! They are often on call and must sleep at the hospital. Why? The system was set up that way and no one has been able to change it.

The Federal Aviation Administration certainly does not allow a pilot to fly a plane if they have only slept a few hours in the last two days. Then why would we allow a surgeon to operate on you or another doctor to prescribe a very strong medication that could potentially hurt or KILL you when they have not slept properly in a week!?!
Being very sleepy is the same as being drunk! Your mind does not work well.

True story: I remember an emergency medical doctor that I know recounting that he was so tired during his residency. He said that once he had been on call for two days in a row with no sleep. On the third day, he finally was able to lie down while at the hospital (still on call) and the minute he closed his eyes his beeper alarm went off meaning that he had to get back up and go see a patient that came into the emergency room. He said that he was SO physically and mentally exhausted that he remembered thinking that he hoped that the patient would be dead before he arrived so that the he could go back to sleep! This is not a mean doctor! The system unfortunately can wear them down until there is just nothing left! It is very sad but this is how the system is right now and you MUST understand it.

So try to be nice to your doctors and nurses! Nurses work just as hard as and sometimes even harder than doctors do! Nurses are extremely overworked and underpaid. Remember that people who entered in the field of medicine--doctors, nurses, technicians--see society AT ITS WORST! They are in the profession to help others; they are not usually there for the prestige or money. In fact, many conventional doctors often leave the profession after 10 to 20 years of practicing because of the stress and difficulty that it puts on their lives even though they may financially be very successful. Medicine is a profession where most people only come to you when they need something or have a problem so they are always coming with negative energy and drawing energy out of you! At least in the naturopathic medicine model, most of the time we see people heal.☺ Imagine how sad and depressing it is in the conventional model where most people do not heal and or only maintain a disease or illness☹.

My mechanic visits: I took my car to my mechanic a few different times. At each visit, I took note of how long the repair time lasted. By the way, at my mechanic I can watch them while they are working on my car. Here are the examples:

- **Oil Change**→took 20 minutes to 45 minutes because he had to check all hoses and the oil flow since oil is very important to the engine working.
- **Change 4 Tires**→took 45 minutes to 2 hours because he had to check each tire pressure, rotate the tires and balance them. Having the wrong tire pressure can pull the car off the road and make me crash!
- **Check Engine Light**→took over 4 hours because he had to check more than 1500 engine codes to find the problem.

Remember, the average doctor's visit is 10-20 minutes or less! I find it extremely sad that in western society our *mechanics have more time to spend with our cars than we give DOCTORS to figure out what is wrong with the body*! Which one is more complex? Obviously the human body!

Now that you have read all the five main issues let us look at this very common scenario:

Scenario: A patient goes to the doctor who *(#5 Does not have enough time)* this→leads to a misdiagnosis or general diagnosis. The doctor prescribes medications based on the symptoms or the name of the disease that the doctor thinks the patient has *(#2 No individualization)*→The medications cause side effects or new symptoms because *(#3 Treatments work against nature/the body)*→The new symptoms are probably in a different organ/area so the patient is sent to a *different* type doctor/specialist *(#1 Emphasis on specialization)*→who prescribes another medication based on his specialty organ/area. The second doctor does not have time to talk to the first doctor. The patient is now on at least two medications from the two different doctors *(#4 Polypharmacy)* →the medications begin interacting with each other and causing more symptoms and problems so the patient has to go back to the same and or NEW doctor(s) and the cycle begins again! Do you see how this is a vicious circle?!

TIPS TO HELP YOU HELP YOUR DOCTOR
You see now that conventional doctors and nurses are very busy so when you go to the visit you can help them by giving as much information as possible, as fast as you can, so that they can arrive at the proper diagnosis.

What doctors typically ask or want to know
Doctors are trying to solve a "mystery" or puzzle of what is wrong with you based on clues that you give us. *Analogy: babies cry for many reasons so you must figure out why it is crying. You mentally go down a list of things right? Usually you think first about the diaper, then hunger/thirst, too hot/too cold, baby is sleepy, baby needs to be burped, baby wants to be held, or baby is in pain...anyway you go down the list eliminating items until the baby stops crying.* Doctors do the same thing when you come in with a symptom! Therefore, you should already have the answers for them when they ask you questions to try to find the problem. If they do not ask you all these questions then you should offer the information! I will give you an **example below**.

Questions they should ask you and how thoroughly you should answer:
- What is the **problem**?—Chest pain
- When did it start?—2 days ago in the afternoon at the family barbecue
- Is it the **first time** you have ever had chest pain like this in your life?—Yes
- Where does it hurt exactly?—In the middle *(point to the area)*
- What were you doing when the pain began?—Sitting at the family barbecue
- What did you do differently a day before the pain started?—I went jogging.

- What does the pain feel like?—It is sharp as if a knife is stabbing me
- How **intense** on a scale of 10 (10 is worst) is the pain?—It is 7-8 over 10.
- Is the pain always level 7-8/10 intense or does it change?—Always 7
- How often does the pain come?—It comes and goes every 2-3 hours
- How long does the **pain last** once it begins?—It lasts 10 minutes
- Does the pain stay in your chest or does it move?—It goes to my arm too
- Do you get **other symptoms** with the chest pain?—Dizziness and sweaty
- What makes the chest pain better?—Lying back in my chair
- What make the chest pain **worse**?—Leaning forward to pick up something
- Has anyone in your family had chest pain?—My dad. He had a heart attack.
- Did you take anything to try and make it feel better?—I took Aspirin
- Did the Aspirin/item you took **help**?—Yes. Decreased pain from 7/10 to 3/10 for about 1 hour but then the pain returned just as strong as before.
- Did you go and see any other health care professionals about this?—No
- Do you have any **health problems** or medical diagnoses?—High blood pressure and Diabetes
- Do you take any **medications or supplements**?—Yes. *Be sure to have a list of meds and supps with doses, how often you take them, how long you have taken them and the reason you are taking them.*
- Do you have **allergies** to any medications?—Yes. Penicillin. It gave me a rash and I had difficulty breathing.
- When did you last have **blood work** done?—A year ago. All normal.

Last doctor visit tips

Remember that based on the questions asked and the responses you give that you will be prescribed a medication and or sent for imaging (X rays, CT, MRI) to try to figure out what the problem is. Therefore, you want to give them all the information so they can arrive at the proper diagnosis.

- **Speak concisely**—do not ramble on and on about how bad the food was at the family barbecue and how Aunt Bessie does not know how to make potato salad! They are busy. Stay on topic and keep answers short.
- **Be detailed in your answers**—follow the example above
- **Do not lie or hold back information**—if you were doing something stupid right before you got the chest pain, such as taking a street drug or even if you were doing something you think is embarrassing or naughty such as having sex or kissing someone else's spouse or partner you should STILL be honest! The ACTIVITY is VERY important in figuring out the diagnosis. The doctor cannot tell your information to anyone else that is called doctor--patient confidentiality.

Some situations may require the doctor to inform a government third party like with gunshot wounds, diseases that can cause an epidemic or in the event of child or senior abuse. Hence, TELL THE TRUTH! AND DO IT QUICKLY! Doctors know when you are not telling the entire story because the symptoms do not match what you are saying. **We are not morons!** When you lie or withhold the entire truth, you just make us mad because you are wasting our time and we are only trying to help you! Do not be embarrassed or ashamed. Everyone does stupid things. Just spit out the information! Most doctors are trained not to judge you/laugh at you or make you feel badly about what you say. Even if the doctor laughs at you (mean doctor) that is not a big deal. Hopefully, you will never see them again. Your job is to get help! *Analogy: you would not take your car to the mechanic and tell him that the engine is shaking but then not mention to him that you disconnected a few wires while you were trying to fix it!*

- **Do not treat your doctor insultingly or as if they are stupid** — what I mean is that **(1)** patients will often show the doctor something random that they just read on the internet and use that information to "prove" that the doctor is wrong. **(2)** Patients can have a bad attitude and ask doctors why it is taking so long to find the problem and how obviously the doctor did not learn much in medical school. The human body is very complex. **(3)** Or in other cases you the patient may even tell the doctor that you just texted someone and that person--with inferior medical training--does not think that the doctors' diagnosis is correct. **True story**: a patient goes to the emergency room for abdominal pain. The ER doctor tells the patient that they believe it is a problem with one of the internal organs. The patient sends a text message to their cousin (a licensed practical nurse/LPN) who disagrees with the doctor's diagnosis. The patient then tells the doctor that they think that the doctor is wrong because the patient's cousin who is an LPN believes the problem is elsewhere. Of course, the ER doctor is FURIOUS at this comment because the ER doctor has completed 13 YEARS of training compared to the 13 months of training it takes to become an LPN!

Yes, it is true that the internet is a great source of information. However, you still need to be able to filter and analyze that information and for medical issues you need a medical background. Not all the information on the internet is correct. It is also true that doctors can be wrong in their diagnoses therefore you can seek a second opinion or request more testing. Ask in a respectful way.

- **Do not answer your cell phone** and have a conversation—only answer if it is to tell family that you are in the emergency room or doctor's office! This is very rude.
- **Be nice to EVERYONE**—if you are mean to receptionists, nurses or doctors all that will do is make them mad at you and then they may certainly stretch your visit time out by HOURS. This happens frequently at the emergency room or urgent care. Remember the saying **"you catch more flies with honey** *(having a sweet attitude)* **than with vinegar"** *(having a bad attitude)*. Remember that your doctor or nurse may have only slept a few hours in the last 2 days, and only eaten hospital food.☹

Recall that the reason that the five issues exist in the conventional medical model is that most people are trying to use it **OUTSIDE** of what it was *originally* intended. Its strengths are for life threatening situations, trauma and reconstructive surgery. There are <u>NO ISSUES</u> with the system when used *appropriately*.

Example of how the conventional system works well: If you are in a bad car accident and your leg is cut off *(#5 Doctors do not have enough time)* is not a factor here because you want them to work as fast as they can! You can die! We are not worried about misdiagnosis either because it is obvious what the problem is…your leg is cut off! We are not concerned with the fact that everyone is treated the same *(#2 No individualization)* because EVERYONE whose leg is cut off SHOULD be treated the same! Stop the bleeding and reattach the leg if possible! To try to reattach your leg we need a specialist *(#1 Emphasis on specialization)* and an orthopedic surgeon would be the doctor to do the surgery. Moreover, since you are in the emergency room, all necessary specialists will gather there to discuss how to save you. So if your heart was damaged in the accident too then the cardio thoracic/heart surgeon would come down to the same room and all the doctors would be together *literally* standing over you! We need many strong medications *(#4 Polypharmacy)* to try to stop the bleeding and to put you to sleep for surgery. We are not concerned with *(#3 Treatments go against nature/body)* in this case because the body has been OVERWHELMED with this injury and <u>will not be able to recover on its own without help</u>. The body cannot stop this kind of bleeding and reattach a leg by itself.

Do you see how *fabulous* this system is **when used properly**! Wow, what a great thing to have access to such a system. This is why I call it the hammer. Fast and furious action. Fantastic! ☺

Naturopathic Medicine Model

On the other hand, if you were trying to repair your TV then you would NEVER use a hammer right? No. That is when you need a screwdriver: slow, steady and precise to get to the bottom of how, when and where the problem started with the wiring of the TV. That is the naturopathic model. People who have long-term disease need slow and steady.

In the naturopathic profession, in general, we are not yet fully covered by insurance companies therefore, we are also NOT bound by time constraints or protocols and therefore we can truly work freely to get down to the bottom of your problem!

The **beauty of naturopathic medicine** is in its principles: **MATH ALERT!**

- Works with the body's natural efforts to heal itself by finding the true underlying cause(s) of disease.

$$+$$

- Uses treatments that enhance healing and in general do not cause any side effects.

$$+$$

- Patient's whole body is considered, and patient is treated as an individual and the patient learns how to care for their health by observing Nature's 9 Health Laws

$$= \text{A Win} + \text{Win situation! Easy math.} \ ☺$$

DON'T BE DOOMED! HERE'S YOUR HEALTH PROBLEM(s) SOLUTION!

Whether you are healthy and trying to prevent illness or if you have been diagnosed with a serious illness, realize that being sick does increase your risk of harm and potentially death...but it does not mean that you are DESTINED to STAY SICK or DESTINED to DIE because we as humans do not control the timing of death. **For example** just think of all of the soldiers that went off to fight over the last few years in Afghanistan and then in Iraq. All of them were at an increased risk of death with bullets whizzing by and bombs blowing up, having to worry about not just enemy fire, but "friendly fire" which is when one group in the military accidently fires on another group in the same military instead of firing on the enemy group. Even though those soldiers were at an increased risk of death, they did not all die...most of them came home right?

Think about car accidents where the car is completely wrecked; flat as a pancake and we are sure that the driver should have been killed but the driver walks away without a scratch. What about that? *YOUNG PEOPLE CAN DIE JUST AS MUCH AS OLD PEOPLE* AND *HEALTHY PEOPLE CAN DIE JUST AS MUCH AS SICK PEOPLE!* ***We do not control the timing of death,*** **but you can** <u>**choose**</u> **to affect the timing of your health!** Therefore, instead of just folding your hands and doing nothing, WHICH IS A GUARANTEE OF WORSENING OF YOUR HEALTH, CHOOSE to take an active role! ☺

Therefore, you should instead AGRESSIVELY AND CONSISTENTLY try **getting back in tune with ALL of Nature's 9 Health Laws** especially "tidying up your tummy"! In addition, ***use natural therapies*** *that do not mask symptoms and that ARE NOT FIGHTING AGAINST what the body is already trying to do to heal itself.* This is why in general, they are *NOT* causing side effects and damaging other organs/areas of the body--*but instead ARE helping the body to heal a specific area(s) and strengthening and rebuilding the ENTIRE United States of You!*

Maybe some of this information is not completely new to you. Perhaps you actually already knew about some of these health laws before and had made some changes in the past but have gotten out of the habit? Or you have made some recent healthy changes but have let yourself "slide" in a few areas because of different life events? It is normal to occasionally "fall off the wagon" and stray from one or two of the 9 laws but then just pick another "reset point/new start date" and get back on the wagon in your journey to health restoration! Whether or not this information is new to you or you were somewhat familiar with it, make a choice **<u>today</u>** for health!
You can do this!

CHAPTER 8: Yikes! So how do I get back in tune with Nat's 9? Full directions!

Great decision to get back in tune with Nature's 9! Remember though, Nature's 9 Health Laws must be practiced together for <u>optimal</u> health! ***Analogy: Consider a car. All car parts must CONSISTENTLY work together for the car to function perfectly. If one tire is slightly flat, the car might shake while driving. If the windshield wipers do not work, then when it rains you may not be able to see to drive and end up driving off the road into a pit!*** Likewise, it is not enough to practice 5 of the 9 laws and blatantly break or ignore the others since they are **<u>ALL</u>** important to the proper functioning of your body! Sometimes you may not be able to do all nine at 100% but just do your best to do most of them at least at 75%! **You can do this!**

NATURE's 9 HEALTH LAWS

AIR #1
Three minutes or so without this VITAL energy source and we will find ourselves lying on the ground passed out! A few more minutes and we DIE! So this is #1! Most of us breathe so shallowly we only use a small part of our lungs and that is bad because many of the bacteria and viruses that make us sick would die if we used air/oxygen better since they die in the presence of oxygen!

- **Jail time--**if we do not change this: Frequent lung diseases: pneumonia, bronchitis, cough
- **Avoid Jail!**—deep breathing! Slows heart rate, calms your nerves, kills oxygen hating bacteria, and relaxes ALL muscles!
- **How to do it**—breathe in through your nose to a count of 3. Count 1 Mississippi, 2 Mississippi etc. as you are breathing in until you reach 3. Count in your head because it is hard to count aloud AND breathe at the same time. Then breathe out through your mouth to a count of 3. Practice often to get deeper breaths/be able to count longer like up to 10. The breathing in and breathing out is one cycle. Try for 10 cycles minimum a day. Then work your way to 30 cycles minimum or more. You can do this as often as you like throughout the day--at work, school, in the car or wherever! It helps the body handle stress. It is great for when your boss or parents just yelled at you.☹

WATER #2

60-80% of our body is made up of water: muscles, bones, blood, organs EVERYTHING! Seven days without it in any form and we die! Most of western society is constantly dehydrated/does not have enough water! Water helps our body throw out trash—solid and liquid—via defecation/pooping, urination/peeing and perspiration/sweating. So if we do not drink enough, we keep trash/wastes in the body and that is a recipe for illness! *Analogy: What if you never took the trash out from your house from week to week for years on end. Think of how dirty your house would be, and the vermin it would attract like rats, cockroaches and other bugs. Gross!* ☹

- **Jail time**—constipation and other digestion problems, stiff muscles, high blood pressure, sticky blood (causes traffic accidents!)
- **Avoid Jail!** —drink plenty! Relaxes muscles and thins out blood.
- **How to do it**—drink about half your body weight in ounces* so if you weigh 100 pounds drink 50 ounces or 6 cups daily—that is a minimum. If you are in a hot environment or are exercising, drink at least 2 cups more. The best types of water are alkalinized or distilled water. But if unavailable or too expensive, do not worry about the type of water JUST DRINK enough! **Note:** the standard measure of a cup is 8 ounces or 250mL. *However if you have a medical condition that requires water restriction check with your physician first.*

BONUS: WHAT ABOUT WATER FILTERS?

In a developed country like the US, we clean the water so that it is not too dirty, like water is in underdeveloped countries. However, filtering water is still a great thing to do since we know that water can contain bad "bugs" like viruses and bacteria, prescription medications (that people flushed down the toilet) also dangerous halides like chlorine and bromine and many other bad chemicals like insect and or weed killers. So what kind of filter should you get? You have to consider six different things: how well it filters, how fast it filters, water waste, pH, installation and cost.

The three <u>most important things</u> to consider are how well it filters, pH and cost.

(1) How well it filters has to do with <u>how many</u> microorganisms (virus, bacteria) or bad chemicals it filters as well as <u>how much</u> it gets rid of these things...meaning cleans out ALL of them or only cleans the water a little bit.

(2) The pH has to do with how acidic or how basic a liquid is. The pH range is from 0-14. The normal pH in your blood is around 7.2 so we like to keep it close to that. Factors like food, water, chemicals and illness can lower the blood pH and make it more acidic which is bad because a lot of "bugs" like bacteria prefer a more acidic environment to grow/multiply in and they can make you sick much faster if your body pH is too acidic. **Analogy:** *you can think of pH as being like a range between two things. So if you are eating food you do not want it to be too sweet (acidic—pH is below 7.2) nor do you want your food to be too salty (pH is basic-above 7.2) you want it to stay more or less in the middle.*

(3) Cost is important obviously, because you have to be able to afford it!

Here is a table that compares some of the most common brands so that you can easily see how they work. The asterisk* is information about filtration time, water waste and installation.

Filter Type and Brands	Filtration quality/removes	PH	Cost
Carbon Filters	poor/ some metals and chlorine	7.2	$50 or less

Brita, Pur and refrigerator filters
Filtration: immediate; Water Waste: none; Installation: none

5 Stage Reverse Osmosis	excellent/ nearly EVERYTHING	4	$100-$400

Kenmore, US Water Systems, Pelican
Filtration: immediate; Water Waste: very high—2 liters of waste per 1 liter purified; Installation: difficult: requires a water line, waste water line and a large space. This process removes all good minerals from the water too. This "empty" highly acidic water can pull minerals from your bones and body ☹ This can be DANGEROUS! To overcome this you would need to add 20 drops of a trace mineral supplement into 2 liters of water. Also, squeeze one whole lemon into 2 liters of RO water to increase acidity. After doing those two things RO water is the cleanest and least expensive option!

Carbon Block Gravity	good/ bacteria and other microbes	7	$250-$600

Berkey, ProPur, AquaCera
Filtration: VERY slow-add water a day in advance; Water Waste: none; Installation: none: requires a large amount of vertical space. Some are portable and can filter any water even from lakes or streams and so these could be useful for camping/rural environments or survival situations. Basic models do not remove fluoride or arsenic so purchase the special filter required for that function.

Distilled Water Purifiers	very good/ all "bugs" & most pesticides	4	$500-$800

Barnstead, Waterwise, Tuttnauer
Filtration: slow--water must be boiled and condensed multiple times; Water Waste: very high 5 liters wasted for every 1 liter purified; Installation: none: requires electricity. Still have to add lemon and minerals like with the RO water.

Dr. Megan uses Nikken Brand[22] Pi Mag Waterfall and Pi Mag Sport Bottle

The Sports bottle is around $50. It filters about 2.5 cups/625 mL. It filters and makes the water slightly alkaline by using multiple layers and magnets. You can take it anywhere and filter water! I used it on vacation with friends and while no one else could drink the disgusting cruise ship water I was fine! ☺ The Pi Mag Waterfall sits on the counter and costs about $400. Both require changing the filters every few months. You can always start with the personal Pi Mag Sport Bottle as I did, and then work your way up to whichever system you prefer!

OK SO WHICH WATER FILTER DO I GET?

-If you want **decent filtration in a ready to go bottle** then the Nikken

-If you want **great filtration at a low price** the 5 Stage Reverse Osmosis is best.

-If you want **good filtration, ease of use and to be able to take it on trips** then gravity filter is best.

-If you need to **get rid of all bad "bugs"** (viruses, bacteria and parasites) or if you live somewhere with no water treatment then the distiller is best.

For more information on water filters and other natural health information see the National Health Advisory website.[37]

NUTRITION #3

Depending on the amount of fat we have on our bodies, we can live at least 3-6 weeks or so without any food at all before we die. However, this law is HUGE since it is the one law that we break the worst and the most often! Healthy nutrition can help the body restore health to itself while a poor nutrition plan actively contributes to a person developing many different illnesses! Numerous studies have been done in different institutions such as schools or even prisons, which clearly show how switching from an unhealthy diet to a healthy diet GREATLY changes ability to learn, and improves behavior...notably less violence amongst prisoners in the prison situation.

   Story: *Before I became a doc, one of my jobs was as a waitress. I used to have to get up early to be at work at 6am, stand on my feet the entire day until 4pm. They would pay me cash weekly. So the energy I put in to get up super early and go to work every day was worth it because I would get paid at the end of the week. One time though, I worked ALL week, getting up early, on my feet and then at the end of the week, they paid me $400 in cash and I put the money in my pocket and left work to go directly to the bank. When I got to the ATM to deposit the cash, I reached into my pocket and the money was not there! I searched frantically in the car, I even drove all the way back to work and walked the* sidewalks and market areas but of course I did not find the money. Well you can imagine how I cried. ☹An entire week of energy wasted because in the end, I had NO money! This is an example of exactly what happens when we eat food that has no nutritional value for us. We have to spend our body's energy in Digestion city making five different organs and three parts work hard to break down the food but then we have nothing to show for it at the end!

Now consider this **fake example:** *What if I had gone to work that same week, getting up early, running around all day...but then while at work I slip on some water and break my leg! Let us say that the company does not pay me worker's compensation, NOR do they even pay me for working that week! That would be awful right? This is an example of what happens when we eat <u>unhealthy</u>* food. Not only do we **spend energy** to break it down/digest it, and we **get NO benefit** from the food (like not being paid), but on top of that, because it is bad food, **it actually HURTS us** (slipping and falling on the job)! Do you see how this works? How often do you think YOU would go to work under those conditions? Not long right? It would be better to just stay at home and do nothing! That is why it is so important to eat well! By the way, most food is either GOOD or BAD! BLACK or WHITE! There really is no GREY! The only food that is neither harmful nor helpful would be ice burg lettuce, which has no nutritional value. It is like water it does not use much energy from your body to break it down.
But anything else you put in your mouth is EITHER helping you, or hurting you!
Then to figure out how much the food/drink is helping or hurting you depends on the amount you eat, when you eat it, and with what other foods you eat it.

Your digestive system is like the "engine of your car" so any problems here are MAJOR! Eating out too frequently—especially fast food or restaurant food-- is a bad because often too much sugar and or salt and other unhealthy colors and additives are in the foods. If you do eat out frequently because you cannot cook *(please do not burn down the house!)* or because you do not have time/resources and must eat out, choose establishments where healthier options are available like Subway Sandwiches, Thai Food, and Buffet places where you can get lots of vegetables.

Note: on the other hand, do not become too crazy and over analyze foods and refuse to eat ANYTHING or eat a very restricted diet for no reason! People who eat specialized or restricted diets are in danger of lacking certain vitamins and minerals. For example, Vegans--people who eat no animal products--are often low in Vitamin B12 and in the mineral Iron, which are found highest and in the best forms in animal foods. In that case, they should first test their levels of these two nutrients and then if they are low, they can take the respective supplements.

Diet note continued: So before you adopt a specialized or restrictive diet, be sure to do your homework about possible nutrients that you may lack or need to supplement if you continue that diet. Read more about vitamins and minerals in the guide later on in this chapter. You can see chapter 17 for more information about supplements and chapter 19 for more information about non-conventional testing.

Jail time--Diabetes, Heart diseases, and many Cancers. YOUR WHOLE BODY IS AFFECTED BY YOUR NUTRITION PLAN!
Avoid Jail!—control your eating and eating environment!
How to do it—my formula is W2H2- **what** you eat, **when** you eat, **how much** you eat, and **how often** you are eating:

- **WHAT YOU EAT:** Home Cooked 5 of 7 days a week so that you can control what is in your food; FRESH FOODS—rule of thumb is fresh foods--like from the veggie/meat/fruit sections--are <u>best</u> and better than frozen foods, and then frozen foods are better than canned foods. Canned foods tend to be very high in salt and also sugar. The lining of the can very often has chemicals that can be harmful to your body and linked with causing cancer. VARIETY: the same way you get tired of watching the same movies, playing the same video games, listening to the same music or whatever, your body gets tired of the same foods! This can potentially lead your police/immune system to get confused and attack those foods causing food allergies and eventually disease! So do not eat the same meals day after day, for weeks on end! **For example,** let us say breakfast is cereal with raw nuts and fresh fruit and dinner is chicken or tofu with spinach and carrots. You really like how it tastes so you ate it one week and then cooked it again the second week. By the third week, you need to switch things! Breakfast can be 2-3 boiled eggs or omelet with avocado and then dinner can be steak or beans if vegetarian/vegan with broccoli and corn. You understand?

    - Eat more **fresh!** Salads and TONS of dark green veggies! Eat twice as many vegetables than you do fruit.

- Colorful: red, green, purple! Try to have all meals with at least 3 colors on the plate and one of them is green—*veggies provide vitamins and minerals and health building stuff—remember this* **fun rhyme to use whenever you are eating, at home, at the buffet or anywhere: *"Yellow and Brown make me frown☹, Red and Green keep me clean!"*** NEVER have an entire plate with all yellow or brown cooked food—like corn, meat, macaroni and cheese, and a baked potato. Your plate should always have at least three colors! Of course, if you ever do want to have just one color let it be green—broccoli, green beans, spinach etc. ☺ Otherwise, try for a minimum three colors. An example plate: carrots, a green veggie, a meat or beans/tofu if vegetarian/vegan. Think rainbow plate. ☺

- **Raw nuts** are a great source of protein! All kinds! Examples: Walnut, Hazelnut, Brazil nut, Almonds, Pecans, Sunflower seeds. Limit Cashews, Peanuts and Pistachio since these nuts can harbor mold on their bodies which can sometimes cause problems with some people. But you can eat them a little bit. *My favorite nut is Pistachio!*
- **Beans** are another great source of protein! Fresh is best meaning that you cooked them from bags versus frozen or canned beans.

- **Limit the amount of animal based foods you eat.** They are much harder to break up/digest and can come from sick animals. Often healthy animals are fed hormones or antibiotics to make them fatter and easier to sell. So remember the formula 70:30. For any meal that has animal based products in it try to make it 70% non-animal foods (like beans, nuts, veggies, grains) and 30% animal based food like meat, fish, dairy--any product from a cow like milk, creams, butter--or eggs. *If it is easier for you to just pick 3 out of 7 days to eat animal products and not eat them the other days than you can do that or you can use the formula with each plate, just make it work for you.*

o If you eat meat, try to eat the **healthiest types of meats**. So among red meats: bison/buffalo or lamb would be better than beef. Among fish deep-sea fish like Wild Alaskan Salmon. Avoid eating meat daily. 2-3 times a week is usually enough. If you must eat meat daily, eat small portions of meat 1-3 ounces. Three ounces of meat would be roughly the size of a deck of cards or a bar of soap.

o **Avoid shellfish**—lobster, shrimp, crab. These bio magnify dangerous chemicals. **Example:** if they eat 2 grams of mercury, they multiply it in their bodies and when you eat it, you eat 4 grams! This is bad because mercury is a very unhealthy/toxic thing often found in the water that destroys especially Brain city!

o **Avoid other seafood** like mussel/clam, shark, and eel because these meats are VERY difficult for the system to digest.

o *Avoid fast foods, fried foods, junk/vending machine foods* most of the time. Eat these foods MAXIMUM once or twice a week and in very small portions.

o **Avoid sweetened beverages** (soda/sweet tea) **and caffeinated beverages**. Caffeine is a stimulant drug. Meaning it "lifts you up" but then it makes you "crash" lower than what you were before you drank it! Plus, it makes both Heart and Liver cities work very hard. ☹ If you must drink sweetened or caffeinated beverages, then drink them MAXIMUM once or twice a week. If you like to drink fruit juices, try for maximum once a day, 8 ounces or less. Get the juices made from fruit only/**not** made from concentrate and without added sugar.

o **Every week or every two weeks** pick one day where you just eat raw foods or just steamed green veggies, fruit and nuts...so it gives your system a "mini" vacation from breaking up heavier foods!

- **WHEN YOU EAT:** You do not want to work hard all day and then just when it is time to leave work and you are tired and ready to go home, your boss comes in and says you MUST stay late and do 2-3 extra hours of work! Your digestive system does not want to work late at night either after a long hard day, while the rest of your body prepares for sleep. Stop ALL eating minimum 3 hours before bedtime. If you are hungry at bedtime, eat a fruit ONLY. It should not take too much time for your system to work on it.

- **HOW MUCH YOU EAT:** eat until you feel slightly full-NOT STUFFED! The crunchier your food is the better--like carrots compared to spaghetti. A lot of chewing sends a signal to the brain that you must be full and so you will eat less. Always try to have a healthy crunchy food in a meal: raw veggies, nuts and apples work well. This is great for two reasons, because in general healthy foods are crunchy and you will also eat less and potentially maintain/lose weight!

- **HOW OFTEN YOU EAT:** Do not eat all day! Your digestive system is five organs/cities. Three of them are the **stomach, small and large intestines.** EACH of these organs is **made of muscles**...just like the muscles of your legs. **Example:** what if I made you go to the gym and run/walk on the treadmill from 7am until 11pm without ANY breaks...you would become very tired right? Think of your poor stomach and intestines working all day long for you in this common *scenario: 7am--breakfast, 9am--beverage, 12pm--lunch, 3pm--snack, 6pm—dinner, 8pm—after dinner beverage—9pm—bedtime cookie.* Your digestive system will now have to continue working EVEN AFTER YOU GO TO SLEEP and likely work until 11pm. So Digestion city has worked from *7am until 11pm* in this scenario with NO BREAKS! Could you last on the treadmill that long? Even walking at a slow pace? Probably not! So eat 2 or 3 evenly spaced, balanced meals a day. Avoid snacking. Allow an hour or two between meals-when no food or beverage is consumed, except for water, so that the system can work—and then REST—before the next meal arrives. *If you have a medical condition that requires a specific diet then be sure to check with your physician first.*

- **Conditions to eat under**: do not eat a full meal if you cannot completely relax and focus on your food. Meaning avoid eating while: working at your desk, while driving, while standing up or while walking somewhere in a hurry! This creates a mix of signals and your body does not know if it should be in "rest/relax mode" or "fight/flight mode" and this will cause poor break down of your food! So if you are very busy with work and must eat, eat a light snack: nuts and fruit, instead of a heavy meal, and that way you will not be starving but at least you will not eat a meal that will not break down well. Even if you only have 5 minutes to eat, try to turn your chair from your work and look at your food and NOT at work! Eat seated and not standing or in motion. Usually, depending on our job/schedule, if we would just properly organize our time, we would not have to eat under poor conditions!

Food preparation and cooking directions:
- ***AVOID DEEP FRYING FOODS***---*high heat and overcooking can "kill" many essential vitamins and nutrients!*
- ***AVOID MICROWAVING FOODS!*** ---Do not COOK food in the microwave just use it to reheat. Use for 2 minutes or less if possible! Using the microwave more than 1 minute already begins to destroy healthy vitamins; *microwaves can "kill" nutrients!*
- **Steaming veggies is best!**--Vegetables are to be LIGHTLY steamed; they should still be somewhat crunchy. Veggies should NEVER melt in your mouth; you should have to chew them! The only reason to overcook veggies is if you have no teeth or weak or fake teeth! ☹
- **Stir frying is second best**---lightly stir fry the veggies in a tablespoon of healthy oil and water until the veggies change color---*high heat "kills" nutrients!*
- **Baking of foods**---baking at temperatures lower than 300 is best—*high heat "kills" food!*
- **Oils*:** Use Olive, Sesame, Coconut and other healthy oils. Avoid Canola, Corn and Palm oils. *Read labels for foods with partially hydrogenated oils.*
- **Seasonings:** Mediterranean sea salt, any FRESH herbs, garlic, cayenne pepper.

*Note: a partially hydrogenated oil is a Trans fat and unhealthy. Avoid!

The idea is to make consistent little changes to your nutrition, so that over time you will eat 90% healthily and 10% unhealthily. In doing so you can still have some "bad" foods that you just LOVE but it will not be a big deal since most of the time you eat well! ☺

HEALTHY MEALS RESOURCES

If you hate cooking and grocery shopping as I do—and you cannot force yourself to do them as I do--then both Fresh N Fit cuisine[71] and Plan to Plate[72] are great short-term or long-term options! Read more about them in chapter 11 "Doc help me lose weight" in the weight loss and healthy meal resources section!

SUGAR THE SWEET KILLER

The body requires a certain amount of sugar to maintain function. The most important natural form of sugar to the body is **Glucose**. All foods will have some type of glucose in them--or after you break down the food, via digestion, glucose is made. It is the main source of energy for the cells of the body, especially Brain city and the red blood cells/semi-trucks. The brain uses approximately 140 grams/day and the red blood cells use approximately 40 grams/day. **Therefore, the body is able to make glucose and put it into the blood/highways. However, that takes energy and it is simply easier to eat food and get glucose that way.** Typically, there is ONLY between 4-8 grams of glucose circulating in the blood at a given time. *IMAGINE how imbalanced the body can become when a person drinks a can of soda, for example, which can have 20-48 grams of sugar!*

Fructose is another naturally occurring sugar (usually in fruits) that is then processed/transformed chemically and then added in high amounts to cookies, cakes, candy--**but even to foods that do not taste sweet-like bread and green beans**. Since it is SWEETER than glucose, fructose has a longer shelf life, and is cheaper. Other names for fructose: corn syrup/solids, high fructose corn syrup. *Remember, sugar in <u>fresh fruit is not processed</u> and is healthy! However if you have blood sugar control issues like Diabetes, even fruit will be a problem.*

The harmful effects of processed sugars on the body systems are numerous and include but are not limited to the following:

- **BRAIN/CENTRAL NERVOUS SYSTEM: (1)**"foggy thinking"**(2)** headaches **(3)** insomnia

- **HEART/CARDIOVASCULAR SYSTEM: (1)** high blood pressure--makes blood "sticky" and harder for the heart to pump around **(2)** pro-oxidation means it damages blood vessel lining/breaks apart your highways **(3)** increases lipids/cholesterol release into the blood/highways→high cholesterol→ increase of illnesses such as a heart attack, stroke, kidney disease, erectile dysfunction and many others.

- **DIGESTIVE SYSTEM: (1)** slows digestion of foods→ can cause diarrhea, bloating, gas **(2)** pulls out minerals--notably copper, chromium and zinc-leading to many illnesses due to lack of essential nutrients **(3)** can lead to Insulin resistance which means the body does not recognize that it needs to take glucose into the cells via insulin→Diabetes **(4)** with regard to satiety/feeling full, the body does not recognize fructose as readily as it does glucose thus it can lead to an increase in the "keep eating" hormone Ghrelin→contribute to excessive eating→weight gain **(5)** the liver processes fructose and this can lead to a buildup of fat in the liver, slowing down its function dramatically.

- **IMMUNE SYSTEM:** slows down the functioning of the immune system. Some studies show that *sugar can significantly decrease the functioning from 2-6 hours!* This is a very serious problem when we think of certain illnesses that require the immune system to be on high alert such as infectious illness (cold, flus) and chronic/ long-term illness such as cancer for example.

- **ENDOCRINE SYSTEM:** can affect hormonal function leading to imbalances notably in the thyroid, pancreas and ovaries.

- **BONES & MUSCLES/MUSCULOSKELETAL SYSTEM:** can lead to a buildup of fat in the various regions of the body—fat cells are typically where harmful environmental toxins, such as mercury, are stored which means we have more areas full of toxins/trash!

Processed sugars are extremely addictive—studies done on **rats in a maze,** showed that rats exposed to both sugar and cocaine **returned to the "sugar water" repeatedly,** almost completely *IGNORING THE COCAINE!*
Beware of "hidden" added processed sugars in: juices, coffee, salad dressings etc.

Note: Many often worry about eating too much salt. No one thinks about eating too much processed sugar. **Excess sugar is 10 times worse than excess salt!** Sugar is the devil.☹ Therefore, if you must pick between salty and sweet, pick salty because a **"sweet tooth" will kill you MUCH faster than a "salty tooth"**! You will not over salt your food or in general, eat food that you think tastes too salty but people can eat high amounts of sugar with no problem! ☹

Remember these other names for sugar: corn syrup/syrup solids, high fructose corn syrup; if it ends in "ol": sorbitol, malitol, xylitol. Definitely avoid artificial sweeteners since these actually "trick" your body because they do not look like normal sugar and so you eat more of this fake sugar than you want to because they are wearing a "mask/disguise" that says to your body "I am not sugar".

Now, in understanding the effects of processed/table sugar on the body, this knowledge can hopefully help you make daily choices to greatly reduce its consumption so that we can continue to create health! Eat less than 20g/day!

BONUS: VITAMIN AND MINERAL GUIDE

Do you know what all the vitamins and minerals are or what foods contain them? No? Do not worry! Here is a list that will help you know how to find them and just how much they help the United States of You! Vitamins and minerals can help you alone, but they usually also are used by another element in your body to make that element work. When another element uses them, we call the vitamin a cofactor. *Analogy: If you are trying to hammer two pieces of wood together, the hammer is the element and the nail is the cofactor.*

Man, I am tired of typing vitamin and mineral over and over again. Oh well. ☹

Vitamins and minerals can be in an **active form or inactive form**. The active form is the vitamin or mineral at work in your body. Usually to use the vitamin or mineral properly your body needs it to be in the active form. The inactive form is a storage form and often your body will then change it into the active form whenever you need that vitamin or mineral. *Analogy: If you were a vitamin/mineral the active form of yourself is when you are awake and working/at school. The inactive form of yourself is when you are just sitting around on the couch or sleeping.* If a person has a health problem, they may have difficulty in transforming the vitamin or mineral into the active form. That is why we may often recommend supplements and make sure that the supplement has the active form of the vitamin or mineral.

Vitamins Water Soluble: B1, B2, B3, B5, B6, B7, B9, B12, and Vitamin C

There are water-soluble vitamins and fat-soluble vitamins. The term water-soluble means that the vitamins LOVE to swim in water. Your blood/highways are made of 80-90% water so that is a good place for them to swim! The vitamins drive-or swim along-to all of your cities and do their work. If you take too many water-soluble vitamins, your body does not store them and you will just pee them out as the blood is traveling through Kidney city. **Remember**: that the body does love to recycle useful things and the Kidneys help with the recycling. However, if there is too much of a particular item and we do not need any more of it, the body will throw it away. If the item is water-soluble then Kidney city will throw out the item via pee/liquid trash.

Vitamins Fat Soluble: K, A, D, E

On the other hand, fat-soluble vitamins HATE being in water. Perhaps they do not know how to swim? Therefore, they will try to avoid the blood/highways if possible. However, they do have to get on the highways to travel to other cities that need them so they will often travel in special delivery trucks called Albumin in order to avoid the water on the highways as much as possible.

Analogy: have you tried to mix oil in water? First, the oil drops spread across the surface of the water, but eventually the oil drops will join to become one big oil droplet. Unlike water-soluble vitamins, if you take too many fat-soluble vitamins they ARE NOT peed out since they try to avoid water as much as possible. Instead, they are stored in your fat, which is very oily and has no water. Therefore, you have to be careful not to take too many of the fat-soluble vitamins because they can build up in your body and become toxic/harmful to you.

Note 1: Fat is where we store ANY toxic chemicals or things that are dangerous to us. We do not want the bad thing to be traveling around the United States of You on your highways/blood vessels and damaging multiple cities and areas. To keep you safe, the item is stored away in fat. *Analogy: If you have a gun in your house, you keep it stored away in a cabinet or in a box. You do not keep a gun on the kitchen table or in plain sight where a child or someone else can get hurt with it.* Fat is like a storage box. The only way to remove the toxic/harmful element from the fat is too burn fat via exercise or sauna. Some dangerous items will come out of the fat and temporarily go into the sweat on your skin. Mercury is one dangerous item that can do this to some extent. Another way to pull items out of the fat is by using a special process called chelation. We can chelate/pull items out of the fat using IV (intravenous or needles in your veins) or using supplements that you swallow. Because fat-soluble items try to avoid water as much as possible, they are not peed out, instead they are thrown out via sweating and pooping/solid trash.

Note 2: to properly take fat soluble vitamins (K,A,D,E) into the body you must take them with foods that have fat in them so meats, nuts, avocado, egg yolks. Think "fat needs fat". Similarly, to digest acidic foods like citrus (lemon, oranges) and garlic, you need enough stomach acid. Therefore, think "acid needs acid".

Minerals
Here is the list: Calcium, Sodium, Potassium, Iron, Zinc, Magnesium, Selenium, Iodine, Chloride, Fluoride, Chromium, Copper, Manganese and Molybdenum.

Note: Minerals also have active and inactive forms and can be water or fat-soluble. The minerals that you really must **be careful** about taking too high doses would be Iron, Iodine, Selenium, Copper and Calcium. They can build up in the body and become harmful. If possible, work with a knowledgeable healthcare professional when you are taking supplements. Read more about supplements in chapter 17.

What Foods Vitamins/Minerals are in and How They Help You
Different foods contain different vitamins and minerals. For example, green vegetables are usually all high in the B vitamins. However, most foods have a mixture of many vitamins and minerals. I did not necessarily list ALL the foods that have these vitamins and minerals. I just listed a few to give you an idea. By the way, many vitamins have two names: a name with a number and then a name with letters.

VITAMINS
Vitamin A or Retinol*
Foods: dairy (cow products), bright colored fruits (oranges), green vegetables
What it helps: eye conditions, skin conditions and immune system
This can build up in the system and then it is harmful.

Vitamin B1 or Thiamin
Foods: meats, fish, grains (like rice), and green vegetables
What it helps: energy production, Brain and Heart cities

Vitamin B2 or Riboflavin
Foods: dairy, meat, dark leafy green vegetables, eggs, mushroom
What it helps: energy production, eyes and headaches

Vitamin B3 or Niacin/Nicotinamide
Foods: meats, fish, almonds and other nuts, avocado, whole grain cereals
What it helps: energy production, skin conditions, Brain and Digestion city

Vitamin B5 or Panthothenic Acid
Foods: meats, fish, eggs, cauliflower, nuts, dates, avocado
What it helps: energy production, Heart city, high cholesterol

Vitamin B6 or Pyridoxine
Foods: meats, fish, soy beans, nuts, cabbage, prunes
What it helps: Joints (arthritis), Brain city, Skin city

Vitamin B7 or Biotin
Foods: animal products, nuts, oats and molasses
What it helps: skin, hair, Brain city and sick nerves like with Diabetes

Vitamin B9 or Folic Acid
Foods: dark leafy greens, beans, eggs, beets, asparagus
What it helps: make DNA (genetic info)—so needed for EVERYTHING! Brain city.

Vitamin B12 or Cobalamin
Foods: mainly animal products (meat, fish, eggs etc.)*
What it helps: Heart city (red blood cells and anemia); Brain city (movement)

Vitamin C or Ascorbic Acid/Ascorbate
Foods: dark leafy vegetables (have more than oranges!), oranges/grapefruit
What it helps: slow wound healing, immune system, skin and bones

Vitamin D or Calciferol*
Foods: eggs, fish and dairy; can also be made in the body via skin and sunlight*
What it helps: bones, autoimmune diseases (body attacks itself), tons more stuff!
This can build up in the system. To make Vitamin D from sunlight includes both Kidney and Digestion cities so if you have a problem in one of these areas--whether you have symptoms or not--you probably will not be able to make this! Vitamin D production also depends on the season, and the position of the earth in relation to the sun. Meaning that being in the sun does not guarantee that you are making Vitamin D. Additionally, remember that the darker skin you have the longer you need to be in the sun. Caucasian/Whites and Asians need minimum 20 minutes while Latinos or African Americans/Blacks need minimum 45 minutes.

Vitamin E or Tocopherols/Tocotrienols (alpha, beta, gamma)*
Foods: seeds, nuts, grains, vegetable oils like olive oil, dark greens, eggs
What it helps: Heart city, Reproductive city (period problems) and Skin city
This can build up in the system.

Vitamin K or Menaquinones/Menadione*
Foods: darky leafy green vegetables, eggs
What it helps: bones, clotting diseases (where you bleed too easily)
This can build up in the system.

All these names and numbers are so annoying. Why did we skip from Vitamin B3 to Vitamin B5? What happened to B4? **Who came up with this system?!?** ☹

MINERALS
Fortunately, the minerals only have names and no numbers! ☺

Boron
Foods: vegetables, fruits and nuts
What it helps: bones and joints

Calcium*
Foods: green vegetables, dairy products, tofu
What it helps: Heart city, Brain city, Musculoskeletal city (bones & muscles)
Taking too much of this in supplement form--especially if not well balanced by other vitamins like Vitamin D and Magnesium--can make it build up in the system causing heart problems and even kidney stones. It is best to get it from eating a healthy diet full of dark leafy green vegetables. If you are taking it in a supplement form, make sure that it has the proper mix of other elements you need. Calcium also requires enough stomach acid to take it into the body properly.

Chromium
Foods: beef, molasses, whole grain breads/cereals, cheeses
What it helps: Heart city, blood sugar control

Copper*
Foods: nuts, poultry (chicken and turkey), dried beans, soy, mushrooms
What it helps: Digestion city (both divisions: digestion and immune system)
This can build up in the system.

Fluoride
Foods: not found in many foods: black tea, seafood. Toothpaste (do not eat!)
What it helps: bones and teeth

Iodine*
Foods: kelp, fish, eggs. Iodized salt.
What it helps: Thyroid county! He helps growth, Digestion city and much more!
Too much or too little of this can destroy Thyroid county!

Iron*
Foods: meats, nuts and seeds, kelp, molasses, prunes and dark leafy greens
What it helps: Red blood cells/semi-trucks! (Heart city), Energy!
Iron can build up in the system. Has good and bad (constipating) forms. Work with a QUALIFIED health professional if supplementing with this. It is very common for people to be deficient in iron or to have enough but not use it well.

Magnesium
Foods: green vegetables, rice, nuts, soy and wheat
What it helps: Heart city, Musculoskeletal city (bones and muscles)

Manganese
Foods: rice, rye, barley, spinach
What it helps: blood sugar problems, nerve problems (Brain city)

Molybdenum
Foods: meats and leafy vegetables
What it helps: joints, bones and muscles (Musculoskeletal city)

Potassium
Foods: fruits, dark leafy green vegetables, potatoes, seeds and nuts
What it helps: Heart city, Musculoskeletal city

Selenium*
Foods: Brazil nuts, garlic *(I am a garlic fiend! I just love it!),* fish
What it helps: detoxing body/cleaning out trash, Thyroid county, immune system
*Can build up in the system.

Silicon
Foods: high fiber foods like grain cereals
What it helps: bones

Sodium
Foods: Prepacked/prepared food is OVERLOADED with this! You don't need a list. ☹
What it helps: Brain city. Seriously, NO ONE lacks this. Eat less prepared foods!

Vanadium
Foods: fish
What it helps: blood sugar problems

Zinc
Foods: nuts, grains, egg yolks, meats
What it helps: immune system, Brain city, skin and a bunch more places!

Whew! Finally finished with that section! I hope that you can see now why it is important to eat many different foods because different foods carry different elements. Having too strict of a diet is not good. However, did you notice how many times I mentioned GREEN VEGETABLES? That is why I have a saying *"Yellow and Brown make me frown ☹ but Red and Green keep me clean"* ☺. Green vegetables are powerhouses of vitamins and minerals so eat them! Remember not to overcook them or to drown them in butter and oil, as is the custom, particularly in the southern part of the United States. ☹

NOTE: many prescribed medications and over the counter drugs can leach or pull these vitamins and minerals out of your body! ☹ Be sure to read about that in chapter 13 under the "drugs that steal vitamins and minerals" section.

BONUS: WHAT DOES DR. MEGAN EAT?
People always want to know what I eat so here it is! **I actually HATE COOKING with a passion! ☹ The only thing I hate worse than cooking is GROCERY SHOPPING.☹☹** However, it is SUPER IMPORTANT to know what you are eating and make sure that the food is healthy and the only way to control that is to cook it yourself. Therefore, I usually grocery shop on one day and cook on a different day so that I do not have to do the two things I hate the most in the same day. ☺

I typically **cook once a week**, usually a Friday afternoon or Sunday morning so that I can have food for the entire week and not have to cook every day since I hate it. Because I just **eat two meals a day,** I cook 2-3 different dishes, which allows me to change at least one meal a day. Planning my meals allows me to control what I eat. Also, I am not "caught" outside hungry or without food and then buy rubbish/junk food.

I wake up between 6am-7am but I do not get hungry until about 3-4 hours later so normally I will **begin the day with liquids**: 3 cups/750 mL of **water**, then I will have 2 cups/500 mL of homemade **veggie juice** (carrot, beets, greens) and then 2 cups of my stress and brain tea. The bulk herbs I use are Ashwaganda, Bacopa, and Eleuthrococcus. *You can learn more about herbs in chapter 15 under the "must have herbs" section.* **I do not have to eat typical western "breakfast foods"** such as cereal, bagels, eggs **at breakfast time**. I usually eat "dinner" foods at breakfast. **TO ME, FOOD IS FOOD, NO MATTER WHAT TIME OF THE DAY IT IS!** I LOVE TO EAT! There is a saying *"Some eat to live, and others LIVE to EAT"*! I fall into that last group! Although that does not mean I eat all the time. It just means I love thinking about food and that I enjoy eating immensely. **I eat 85% vegan-no animal products- kosher and gluten free** . I do not have any specific allergies to these food types (believe me I have tested for them) but I feel that this diet helps keep me from eating trash. I do not eat the gluten free cereals/breads/crackers or other products though because they contain rice flour to substitute for the wheat flour and I DO have sensitivity to rice. **I eat very little to no processed sugar.** This is easy to do since I am making 90% of my food myself, mainly from fresh ingredients. I do not add sugar to my cooking, nor do I go out to eat more than once a week. I usually eat with the same pattern for 9 months of the year and then vary my diet slightly during the 3 summer months of June-August so I separated my diet here by summer breakfast and dinner and then what I eat the rest of the year. The approximate times that I eat meals are the same throughout the year.

Summer Breakfast 11am
I tend to eat lighter in the summer months than in the other months so a typical meal for breakfast in summer might be a **smoothie.** My two favorite recipes are identical except you just change which fruit you use. You may need to add more liquid than what I have here depending on what fruit/nuts you use. You want it to be smooth and flow easily. This recipe usually makes enough smoothie for 2 days or so because I drink 2 cups/500mL at a time.

- 2 cups/500 mL almond milk (but you can use water)
- 2 ripe bananas (with brown spots)
- 3 ripe mangos or a packet of frozen mango for "Mango Madness" **OR** 2 packets of fresh berries of any kind or frozen berries for "Berry Blast"
- 2 cups/500mL of walnuts (but you can use any type nut)
- 2 small black avocados.

Blend in the blender. If you use the mango as your fruit, it is "Mango Madness smoothie" or if you use the berries, it is "Berry Blast" smoothie! This recipe gives you enough protein (from the nuts and almond milk), healthy fat (from the avocado) and carbohydrates (from the fruit) to last at least a few hours. You get tons of vitamins, minerals and omega 3s/essential fatty acids! ☺ This is usually my breakfast during the late spring through summer months.

Sometimes I eat **bread** with nut butter (Almond, Peanut or Hazelnut) and apple butter or a sliced banana on top for a little sweetness. I make my own bread using a bread maker I bought at the thrift store for $10. I buy Bob's Red Mill Brand[38] gluten free and dairy free flour and then just put the oil, salt, yeast and egg into the bread machine and it does all of the work! It stirs, lets the mixture sit and rise and even beeps when it is time to add in extra ingredients I might want such as raisins or nuts!

Rarely I eat **cereal** for breakfast—meaning perhaps I buy a box every 6 months or so. The best brand with the least amount of sugar is the **Uncle Sam brand**[39].

It usually has only four ingredients that you can easily pronounce and understand what they are: whole-wheat kernels, whole flaxseed, salt and barley malt. In each ¾ cup serving size there is 10 grams of fiber (helps with pooping); 9 grams of protein which helps keep you full, and almost everything in your body is made of protein; less than 1 gram of sugar; and has Omega 3's or essential fatty acids/EFA. My favorite flavor is the Original Wheat Berry Flakes. I can eat it plain, but I add nuts, dried or fresh fruit for sweetness or even a little raw honey. The milk that I use is either almond or coconut milk. I also use soy, hemp or cashew milks.

However, as I said, typically I eat cooked "dinner" foods for breakfast for 9 months of the year.

Summer Dinner 6pm or 7pm latest
When it is hot outside, I usually want cooling foods and so I will eat mainly salad. Those of you who know me well know how much I **HATE** salad.☹ Yes, it is very healthy for you but to me it is rabbit food. I love cooked food and will eat any vegetable under the sun, but I have always hated salad since my childhood. Nevertheless, in the summer it is cooling so I eat it. I love my food to be colorful, and especially in a type of food that I do not like very much, so I make my salad VERY colorful. I use carrots, dark greens (romaine lettuce or kale), onions, raisins or cranberries for a little sweetness, tomatoes--although I cook these slightly to get the healthy lycopene in the tomato to come out; lycopene only comes out with heat--and beans (any type) for protein.

I make my own salad dressing with Olive oil and sea salt. My favorite dressing is with some Eden French Celtic sea salt or Alessi brand sea salt, 2-3 cloves of crushed garlic, dried dill and dried oregano.

I also prepare **light stir-fry veggies** with beans for protein.

I **rarely eat meat** perhaps once or twice a month—often even less than that. I usually purchase it myself--meaning I very rarely eat meat out at restaurants--to make sure it is a good quality. The only red meat I eat is bison because they are still raised in a healthy, natural environment. Many cows/beef live in the city in stalls! These big animals should be out free roaming grasslands and eating their normal diet of grass instead of other ridiculous things. You can purchase bison in many places but I purchase mine at the Dekalb Farmer's Market. I usually freeze it since I do not consume very much. You can also purchase quality beef there. *Look online for places where you can order healthy meats from natural, local farms.* VERY rarely, I get beef that was grass fed and finished. This means the cows only ate grass and not corn and other stuff that is not normal for them to eat.

I avoid eating animal products with antibiotics or hormones in them. I rarely eat fish just because my body does not seem to like it. However, if I eat fish I only eat deep-sea fish with fins and scales like the Wild Alaskan Salmon brand. On rare occasions, I eat turkey or chicken.

Spring, Fall and Winter Meals

During this period, I eat heavier meals: soups, nut/vegetable loafs, and casseroles. I eat these foods for breakfast and dinner. **This week for example** I am eating a raw nut loaf with vegetables for breakfast and having either a smoothie or a tomato basil black bean soup for dinner. The tomato, basil and black beans were all fresh. I may alternate one meal with the smoothie or with bread and nut butter or an alternative butter like Earth Balance brand fake butter. It is made with Safflower, Flax and Olive oils and spreads on bread like butter.

Snacks

I VERY rarely eat a snack between meals. Maybe once a week. Why? Remember that your digestive system is made of muscles and it is best to work them during a meal and then let them rest an hour or two before the next meal. If you snack between meals, you work your digestion muscles ALL day with no breaks--like you having to jog/walk ALL day with no rest--and it messes up your digestion.
I use snacks in the two following ways **(1)** if I am really too busy working/running around to eat a proper meal seated, eating peacefully and chewing slowly, then I will eat snacks just to give me enough energy until I have time for a full meal **(2)** I use snack foods to replace a meal. **For example**, *the other day I ate my nut and vegetable loaf for a late breakfast around 12pm. I was full for at least 5-6 hours. By 630pm I still was not hungry but I knew I that I needed to eat again because I would be hungry eventually by 730pm which is TOO late for me to eat since I normally go to bed by 10 or 1030 pm. Instead, I decided to eat a snack food.* That is how I use snacks. I tend to prefer salty foods or have a "salty tooth" than sweet foods or a "sweet tooth".

Snacks that I have to prepare or mix in some way:

- **Popcorn**—I get the Jolly Time brand white kernels. I pop it myself on the stove top using olive oil. Then I add sea salt and sometimes pepper and herbs like Thyme.
- **Dark Chocolate with raisins**—I buy the Ghirardelli brand 100% dark chocolate bar and then eat 2-4 squares of it with about 4 pieces of raisins. You see, chocolate is not naturally sweet. They add a lot of sugar to make chocolate sweet! ☹
- **Nuts with dried cranberries**—I eat a handful of mixed or single nuts- Hazelnut, Walnut, Pecan, Brazil, Sunflower seeds-with half a handful of

cranberries. I limit Cashews and Peanuts because they are more likely to harbor mold. But I do eat them sometimes. I usually buy nuts that are raw and unsalted.

- **Smoothies**—again I always have fruit, nuts and avocado in it. Sometimes spices like ginger, nutmeg or cinnamon.
- **Hummus with bread**—hummus is made from chick peas/garbanzo beans. You can buy it or make your own. Sometimes I make my own sometimes I buy it. My favorite flavor is the red pepper flavor.
- **Corn chips and salsa**—I buy Olé corn chips-a Mexican brand that has less salt and additives compared to other brands-then I make my own salsa.
- **Sweet potato fries**—I buy sweet potatoes and then make my own fries by cutting the potatoes into small pieces. I season with salt, turmeric and curry powders. I bake them at about 300 degrees for an hour.
- **Crispbread cracker mini sandwich**—I get the Wasa brand.[40] I start with the cracker as a base and then put on an alternative/fake cheese. I use the Daiya brand.[41] If I use real cheese then it is either French or Swiss from Dekalb Farmer's Market. I use a slice of tomato, avocado, onion and add sea salt and dried dill seasoning. YUM! ☺ I LOVE this cracker because it has no sugar, very low salt and is high in fiber and protein with a few simple ingredients! **Note:** I also eat crispbread with almond and peanut butter and raw honey or crispbread with Earth Balance fake butter and apple butter!
- **Two Hard-boiled eggs**—with sea salt. I look for eggs from chickens allowed to roam freely and fed a vegetarian diet. Chickens raised in cages are not happy. You would not be happy in a cage either. They have high stress hormone, they get sick more often and are pumped with antibiotics. Then we eat their high hormones and drugs! Also, I want a vegetarian chicken. Some farms feed <u>dead</u> chickens to their *living* chickens...and the living chickens will eat the dead chickens. Just seems wrong. You will have to ask a chicken directly why they would eat their fellow brother/sister. ☹ I use Horizon Organic brand.

Store bought snacks/ready to eat
- **Sweet plantain chips**—I buy the Ocho Rios brand[42]. I usually find it at the Jamaican/African/Mexican restaurants or stores. I like them because they are naturally sweet only because the plantains themselves were sweet--no added sugar--and are low in salt. They only have two ingredients: ripe plantains and vegetable oil. They are also very crunchy so I do not over eat them because my jaw gets tired of chewing very quickly! They come in individual size bags and not a big bag so that helps too.
- **Kind brand bar**[43]—I like this because it is only made of fruit and nuts.
- **Ovaltine cookies**—the orange packet cookies. They are not healthy but I love them! They are high in sugar. I may buy a packet three times a year.
- **Candy**—I virtually NEVER eat candy, but if I do, I buy 1 or 2 ginger chews or hard caramels.

Eating at restaurants with healthier choices. _Great book_: **In Defense of Food**[73]
I only do this once a week so that I can control what is in the food I am eating.
My favorites:

- **Thai restaurants** (most often. 3 out of 4 weeks)—I get the garlic stir-fry veggies with tofu, a curry dish or veggie low mein.
- **Subway**—I get the foot long veggie and baked chips. I usually only eat here during summer months.
- **Panera Bread**—the Mediterranean turkey sandwich with chips and soup.
- **Golden Corral buffet**—I get broccoli, green peppers and onions, a little macaroni and cheese, purple cabbage, carrots and hush puppies—these are just greasy bread balls but I love them! I eat two bread rolls as my dessert. I do not get true dessert. I usually eat here only on some holidays.
- **Jamaican restaurant**—I get two veggie patties.
- **Farm Burger**[69]—high quality beef! Good oils for French fries!
- **Other cuisines**: I LOVE TO EAT and I am not picky! I eat African, Caribbean, Mexican/Central/South American, European, Mediterranean, Asian, Indian, Middle Eastern and raw food restaurant cuisines! ☺

Eating at less healthy restaurants/fast food. _Great book_: **Fast Food Nation**[74]
I only do this maybe twice a month or less. Unless I find myself in a bad week where I have not been cooking--because my schedule is crazy--and then I may eat fast food two or three times a week. This only happens every 3 or 4 months though because when I eat badly I FEEL badly very quickly. My body is so used to healthy food that I can only eat unhealthy food a few meals before I begin to feel low energy, joint pains or swelling. My favorites:

- **Taco Bell**—I get two fresco (no cheese or mayonnaise) bean burritos and add guacamole and many onions.
- **Pizza**—I like Little Caesar's $5 hot and ready cheese or Pizza Hut's thin crust with three vegetable toppings: mushroom, onion and spinach.
- **French fries**—McDonald's are my favorite and then Checkers is second best. I just love the salt and warmth!

Beverages
My main drink (99% of the time) is water. I drink half my body weight in ounces so about 6-9 cups. I drink 3 cups first thing waking up in the morning, 3 cups an hour or two after breakfast and then 2 cups after dinner. If the water is in a non-transparent bottle, I may not realize I have not drunk enough as the day is moving along, so I make sure my water is in a clear bottle so that I can see how much I have drank. I do not drink with meals, I drink mainly in-between meals so that I have more room for food ☺. Otherwise, I daily drink vegetable juice that I make with my own juicer and herbal teas that I make from bulk/not in tea bag herbs.

The only **juice** I may drink once or twice a week is the **Simply Brand**. The fruit juice is not from concentrate and has no added sugar. It is only sweet because the fruit in the juice is sweet. I do not use caffeinated beverages at all and maybe once or twice a year I may have half a soda. Root beer or orange are my favorites.☺ By the way, the **juicer** I use is Jack LaLanne's. It costs around $99 dollars and lasts for at least 3 years before you may want to replace parts or buy a new one. I like it because it separates the juice from the pulp or fiber of the plant. I do not like pulp in my veggie or fruit juices. If I am drinking I want to ONLY drink; I do not like drinking AND chewing at the same time.☹ Other ways to make healthy beverages like smoothies, and nut milks at home is to use a **Vitamix**. They are more expensive $300-$400 but you can make ANYTHING in them including food and not just beverages. A **blender** is a nice way to make a beverage too...if you like pulp.

BONUS: DR. MEGAN'S FAVORITE COOK BOOKS
Since I HATE cooking, I try to spend AS LITTLE time in the kitchen as possible. I do not invent or experiment with making my own recipes since that could end in tragedy: either death or dismemberment.☹ Therefore, I rely upon cookbooks. I look for cookbooks with clear instructions, few ingredients, low preparation time, and preferably with pictures! They are typically vegan or vegetarian cookbooks since I barely eat meat. The cookbooks for meat eaters usually make meat the center of the recipe, so buying vegetarian cookbooks I can just add meat if I want to.

- **Classic Vegetarian Cooking** by Linda Fraser
This one is my favorite! Thanks to my beloved sister G for introducing it to me!
- **The Detox Health-Plan Cookbook** by Maggie Pannell
Has recipes and great lifestyle advice too! Thanks to my mandi-kins M.B. for giving it to me!
- **The Pretty Darn Quick Vegetarian Cookbook** by Donna Klein
I found this at the thrift store...I think. It has some vegan recipes too.
- **Garden of Eaden** by Evelyn Lumpkin
This natural master chef and world traveler extraordinaire has a passion for encouraging others to live a healthy lifestyle! Check out her non-profit organization Abundant Life Health Association.[59] Feel free to donate!
- ***S.N.A.C. It Up!*** *by Shi*
*I did not misspell the word "snack"! This is an acronym for **S**hi's **N**atural **A**pproach to **C**ooking". This young lady is only 11 years old and already she is working hard to encourage other young people to eat healthily but also to love and value themselves! Please support her! It is so nice to see a young person who is trying to help others in her age group! Get her book and look for her media events on her website www.snacitup.com! Watch out world, Shi's coming!* ☺

SLEEP #4

A few rare genetic diseases prevent a person from sleeping AT ALL during the night. You can die from a complete lack of sleep. How long it takes can vary between months to years...depending on how severe the illness is in the person. Sleep is very important because that is the time the body rests and restructures. Remember that studies show that after only ONE night of complete loss of sleep or very poor sleep that is equivalent to you being slightly drunk. Yes! Your ability to function, think and react is **_much_** worse! Studies show it can take a few DAYS for you to catch up on one night of poor sleep. You do not catch up simply if you go to bed early the next night! So if you are constantly going to bed late or sleeping poorly then you have a constant sleep deficiency! The amount of sleep we all need varies however; in general, adults need a minimum of 6-10 hours. Remember that the best quality of sleep happens in the hours before midnight; so if possible, try to get to bed at least an hour or more before midnight.

- **Jail time**--poor decision making/performance at work/school; Obesity— some studies show that poor sleep can cause us to overeat; irritability.
- **Avoid Jail!**—set a sleep routine *one hour before bedtime* and try to go to bed at approximately the same time every night **(1)** Turn lights down low in the house. This allows the sleep hormone Melatonin to know that now that it is darker, it is time to make you sleepy. This hormone only comes out in darker settings—so if the house stays bright with overhead lights the body thinks it is still time to say awake **(2)** Put on pajamas **(3)** Avoid any stimulation! No making decisions with your spouse; no stimulating TV shows like violence, politics or comedy. It is time for your body to wind down. Stop all phone calls. You do not want good stimulation--a friend calls to tell you that they got a new job; or bad stimulation—a friend calls to say that they were fired. **(4)** No eating or drinking at bedtime **(5)** Before bedtime make a quick list of items you want to accomplish for the next day, so that you do not lie awake thinking of things to do. However if you are lying in bed and STILL thinking of the next day's events, keep a pad at the bedside table to quickly add items onto the list in case you forgot something. That way you are not lying there worrying if you will remember to do item X the next day **(6)** Go to bed in a dark and quiet room...unless you are afraid or have issues with darkness. Then a little low light is ok.

EXERCISE #5

The phrase that says *"move it or lose it"* is so true here! Your arms and especially your legs are the engine of your heart. The same way you do not want your toilet to become clogged and stop flushing *(ewww!)* we do not want your heart, which pumps blood around your body to become sluggish and exercise keeps this from happening! Also, via sweating we can eliminate many toxins/trash that build up in the body because we are breaking up the fat where these toxins were stored by the body to keep you safe.

- **Jail time--**heart disease: high blood pressure, strokes, and heart attacks. HEART DISEASE IS THE NUMBER ONE KILLER OF MEN AND WOMEN IN THE UNITED STATES!
- **Avoid Jail!**—pick something you like doing so you will not avoid it. Think exercise classes, sports, YouTube videos, dancing to music at home or at a dance spot, outdoor activities when weather permits like hiking, biking; using a mini indoor trampoline at home--you can walk in place on it too if you cannot jump. If possible, get a friend for accountability. It is easy to let ourselves down and quit or not do enough, but it is not so easy to disappoint a friend. Then you can encourage each other! Again, you and your exercise friend do not have to be together to exercise—call them at exercise time and exercise over the phone or computer! You can have an exercise friend in another state or country! Make a goal for yourself...like to exercise a certain amount of times per week and then when you reach your goal give yourself a reward! Probably best if it is not food...so maybe treat yourself to a movie, sporting event or a spa day!

- **How to do it**—aerobic is best*—meaning where your heart is pumping fast and you are sweating because your heart is pumping faster. A routine that has elements of aerobic and non-aerobic would be great. Start small and work up—even 5 minutes a day of just jumping jacks at your house is better than nothing. Remember, *"a little bit of SOMETHING is better than a lot of NOTHING"*! Start with just one day a week for a few minutes then work up to at least 3-4 days a week, 20-30 minutes a day. Remember you can sneak in exercise by walking up and down the steps at a fast pace, over and over, either at work/in or near your house; by parking far away from grocery stores; and you can also do intense intervals. For example 10 minutes of running in place/or just lifting your legs up and down fast or jumping jacks 3 times in the day. You do not have to do all 30 minutes at once! Be sure to stop exercising 2 hours before bed so you do not have your body too excited to calm down to sleep.

If you have a medical condition that restricts movement check with your physician for alternative forms besides aerobic/heart pumping exercise such as isometric exercises where you hold up and out either one or both arms or legs for a few minutes without actually moving them. This works muscles without moving them because the muscles are working against gravity.

GROUNDING: TIME OUT IN NATURE #6

There are so many beautiful and interesting things to see out in nature: sunshine, flowers, trees, animals and insects yet most of us are completely ignoring them! We spend all of our time indoors looking at/working on some form of electronic device-TV, computer, cell phone or other machinery! Studies have shown that those who live in regions where sunlight is low–such as in the northwest of the United States and parts of northern Europe--have significantly higher levels of depression…just from a lack of sunshine! Remember the sunlight on your skin also helps your body to produce vitamin D a super important factor in staying healthy from colds and flus and many other illnesses!

Additionally, since most of us spend almost 24 hours a day inside we are exposed to all the indoor pollutants: viruses/bacteria/dust/mold/industrial toxins that are present in the heating and air-conditioning systems. How often do you think they clean the vents in your school/work place? Most likely is that they never have! Do they have filters to help keep the airflow clean? Probably not! What about in your home? Therefore, there are likely years of dust/infectious organisms and other "trash" that we spend ALL DAY BREATHING, DAY AFTER DAY! Indoor air is highly more polluted than outdoor air—even if you were sitting in traffic behind 100 cars emitting exhaust, the air in your home and work is MUCH more polluted!

- **Jail time--**depression, indoor pollution illnesses such as "sick building syndrome" often causes long-term fatigue and frequent colds/flus.
- **Avoid Jail!**—incorporate fresh air and time outside daily! You can open your car windows while driving to get fresh air, open windows in your home and take a few breaks outside for 5-10 minutes twice a day or so. In the summer if it is super-hot and you must use air conditioning, once it cools down in the evening open up the window in the room where you spend the most time (bedroom or living room) for at least 20 minutes to allow fresh air to circulate. Even in the winter if it is very cold, open up the window at the warmest part of the day and allow air to move in and out. Or you can even leave the window in your most commonly used room open just a crack all day long, to allow fresh air inside. Spend time outside even if just for a few minutes sporadically, or sit near a window and let the sunlight touch your skin for a few minutes.

Remember: The darker your skin the longer you need to be in the sun to produce vitamin D. Review the Vitamin D section a few pages back for details.

POSITIVE MINDSET/SPIRITUALITY #7:

This one is also huge because it involves the control tower of your entire body, which is your mind! *A SICK/UNHAPPY mind can totally make a healthy body sick, just as a sick body can affect an otherwise healthy mind!* That saying **"mind over matter"** is very true! Once a person's mind is full of negative emotions such as fear, sadness, anger, resentment, and worry then it makes the body produce the stress hormone, Cortisol, which in turn causes NUMEROUS health problems when it is constantly high! Therefore, it is very important to keep the mind positive and full of emotions such as happiness, contentment, and thankfulness. It is true that many of us have lived horrible things in life but we must keep moving forward as we work through these things! If you have a religion or spiritual practice, many studies show that these individuals are in general healthier, happier and live longer than people who do not!

Jail time--mental illness, heart diseases (stroke, heart attack), digestion illnesses and cancer!

Avoid Jail! How to do it—(1) Forgiveness—*this may require professional help. Forgive others* for what they did to you—it does not make what they did ok, it just means you can move on with life because they probably already have moved on! Again, holding onto resentment/anger or any negative emotion is like YOU drinking poison and waiting for the OTHER person to die! Also, *forgive yourself* for what YOU may have done to others OR done to yourself and try to make amends!

(2) Live in the present—studies show so many of us live in the PAST or in the FUTURE—thinking things like "in the past I was abused or happier", or "in the future when I have more money I'll be happier", or "I hope I do not get disease X in the future". We are never living in the present! Take this day-here and now- and live it to the fullest!

(3) Thankfulness—it is true that we could complain about things, but remember that someone else's life is MUCH worse somewhere in the world! It does not mean that your problems are not important but wallowing in them for days, weeks or months on end does not change the problem! Allow yourself to be upset about the problem for a specific amount of time—a few hours, a day, a week or month. The amount of time will depend on the gravity of the problem of course, since it is easier to recover from a bad day at school/work than from the death of a beloved person. Then try to find something to be thankful for such as food, a home, relatively good health, friends etc.

Alternatively, be thankful that a bad situation is not worse! Thankfulness allows us to look past the immediate problem. Make a list of things to be thankful for and you may be surprised how much you can find!

(4) Try to create solutions to problems--If there is a persistent problem, then instead of only complaining or being angry/sad, create solutions. Complete or permanent solutions are not always possible immediately. They may take more time: weeks, months or even years to prepare a resolution to the problem. It may involve a job/career change, increasing schooling/education levels, a move, counseling, separation from family/spouse—although hopefully only a temporary separation. Therefore you may not be emotionally, financially or physically able to make the change right now—but if possible, look for a temporary solution and remember to support your health in other ways—healthy diet, sleep etc. while you are going through this hard time.

(5) Surround yourself with supportive people—limit contact with negative people. It may be difficult if they are in your household. If that is the case, then look for emotional support from outside—a coworker, counselor/life coach, health professional, perhaps existing friends, or go to places to make new friends. *Although if you are in a couple, be VERY careful not to compromise your relationship! Often confiding in someone else--like a wife complaining about her relationship with her husband to a male coworker/friend or vice versa--can lead to disaster!*

How to do it BONUS—positive affirmations—use them after ANY negative thought such as *"I am too fat/skinny, too old/young, ugly, dumb. I will never amount to much/I am worthless. I will never be better. No one loves me. My life or health will always be this way"*. IMMEDIATELY follow it with a positive affirmation that states the exact opposite. Speak this aloud if possible! **Do not say it aloud in the middle of school/work because people will look at you funny**. Follow those negative thoughts above with these *"I am working on my ideal weight and will achieve it! I am not too old; I am the age I should be! I am beautiful! I am intelligent and if I want more intelligence, I can achieve it! I am worth more than gold! I can try to become better by putting my resources together and diligently working towards it! There are people that care for me because I am important! My life and health can change because I am working to improve them!"* You must actively practice this while you work on assembling all the necessary elements to make whatever big change you want to achieve. *PRACTICE BEING CONTENT **NOW** AS YOU ACTIVELY WORK TO GET WHAT YOU WANT!*

PURPOSE #8: We all need a reason to get up in the morning! Some studies have shown that many people that enter retirement and then do not maintain an active lifestyle/engage in other activities are significantly unhappier than when they were working and may have more risk for depression and suicide! Think about the celebrities that have tons of money and free time but still feel like their life is useless! Although lying on the couch all day long might be nice for a few weeks, it is not good for health for a long period of time! We need to feel useful in this life. For most, this is work, school or being involved in the community.

- **Jail time--** depression, suicide, heart disease.
- **Avoid Jail!**—look for a cause: a person, organization, or ideal that you can work with to help make it prosper in a positive way! Think adopt-a-grandparent, big brother/big sister, save the environment, community events like gardens etc. Work with people that are more ill/handicapped then you etc. Especially now with the Internet the sky is the limit!

FUN! JUST FOR ME! #9: this has NOTHING to do with purpose or for a reason! It is not for any ideal/individual/job. You do it simply because you LIKE to and because it makes you happy! Find some healthy activity that you enjoy. It may or may not involve other people; it is ok to make time to have fun alone. You are worth it!

- **Jail time--**Mental illness, fatigue, irritability.
- **Avoid Jail!**—could be any activity: outdoor activities, playing with animals, dancing (at home in your living room is ok too!), board games, singing (maybe in the shower if you can't carry a tune in a bucket!), sewing, window shopping, museums...JUST WHATEVER IS FUN FOR YOU! Do this minimum 20 minutes at least once weekly.

You can do this!

NATURE'S 9 HEALTH LAWS CHEAT SHEET!

We discussed many things in the Nat 9 instructions so I have included a "cheat sheet" so that you have only one or two sheets of paper with all of the main instructions on it. There are three levels of participation. **Beginner level:** try to do at least one or two or three of Nat' 9. Do them as well as you can. **Middle level:** try to do between 4 to 6 of any of Nat's 9 consistently. **Advanced level:** try to do all 9 of Nature's Health laws! It would be fantastic if you could do the Dr. Shulze[4] cleansing program(s) that I recommend when you start Nat's 9! See chapter 10 "How liquid fasts help my body clean out trash/detox" for more information.

NATURE'S 9 HEALTH LAWS CHEAT SHEET

NUTRITION OPTIONS: Fresh! Home cooked! Many colors! Green especially. Beans and nuts! Think Fiber and bitter foods! Low animal products! Healthy meats!

THE MAIN IDEAS: *Fresh foods are better than frozen foods, which are better than canned foods.*

(1) Try to eat 2-3 evenly spaced meals with 3-4 hours between meals
(2) Heavy meals at breakfast or lunch; protein and healthy fat at each meal
(3) Light meal or snacks for dinner
(4) Avoid snacking between meals-leave 3-4 hours for digestive organs to work and then rest without anything else new coming in except water
(5) Finish eating 3 hours before bedtime
(6) Do NOT lie down after eating ANYTHING! If you must sleep, sleep upright
(7) Avoid fast food, fried foods, junk/vending machine food
(8) Eliminate hard to digest meats: pork, sausage, ham, and shellfish—can eat beef, bison, turkey, chicken and deep sea wild caught fish
(9) No mixing meats at mealtime—pick one type meat and eat that.
(10) Avoid processed sugar with meals-- natural sugar in fruit is fine-eat a sugary dessert 30 minutes before meals ☺ or 1 hour after meal. If it is only a little cookie that is ok to eat with the meal but no big pieces of cake with frosting or sugary pies though. No high sugar drinks with meals: soda, juices, sports drinks, or milk shakes. Only water. A little juice with no added sugar is ok though. If you must drink a sugary drink with the meal then no more than 4 ounces. Otherwise, on occasion you can drink these sugary drinks in between meals
(11) Eat more fiber: fruits like apples and pears and dark green veggies

Fluids: stop ALL drinking 90 min before bed so you do not disturb sleep to pee.
- **Water intake:** minimum half of your body weight in ounces. *Plain* water. Meaning do not count "tea" or "lemonade" as water!

SUPPLEMENT OPTIONS:

First do Dr. Shulze's 5 Day Bowel Cleanse and then do his 5 Day Liver Cleanse and then you can use these supplements along with the nutrition and home options. *He also has a 5 Day Kidney cleanse you can do. Then restart the cleanses again! His herbs/cleanses are fantastic!* **Try to do one of his 5 day cleanses at least once a month**. *If you cannot afford to purchase the actual Dr. Shulze cleanses, look up the herbs he uses and purchase 2-3 ounces of two to three of them at your local herb stores and do your cleanse that way! The bulk/fresh herbs vary in price but typically cost between $2-$3 per ounce and with two ounces of three herbs total that should cost you approximately $12-$18! That will last you approximately a week!* **Recipe:** *1 Tablespoon of each herb into 1 liter/4 cups of water. Bring to a boil. Turn off fire. Drink two cups of tea daily. Drink hot or cool.*
His herbs/cleanses are better though, so if you can afford it do his programs!

- Genestra Brand Super EFA Liquid (Fish Oil) natural orange flavor
- Genestra Brand HMF Intensive Probiotic
- Designs for Health Brand L-Glutamine
- Klaire Labs Brand Vitaspectrum capsule formula multivitamin

HOME OPTIONS:

You can do deep breaths/ movement/outside time in shorter periods meaning that you can exercise for 10 minutes twice times a day if you wish.

- **Deep breaths daily:** 10 cycles.
- **Movement daily:** 20 minutes minimum.
- **Fresh air and sunshine daily:** 20 minutes minimum.
- **Bedtime*:** by 10-11 pm in full darkness (if you do not fear the dark).
- **Daily alternating shower hydrotherapy**: 4 cycles minimum. *See chapter 15, #2 for more information on this therapy!*
- **Daily Castor oil cloth**: minimum 4 consecutive days over low abdomen for minimum 30 min. *See chapter 15, #3 for more information on this therapy!*
- **Positive Affirmation/Purpose:** I am creating health now! *Or make up one!*
- **FUN (Just for me):** insert your own activity. Do the activity at least once a week for minimum 20 minutes.

**Recall the hours of sleep* <u>*before*</u> *midnight are much better for your body but bedtime depends on your job/school. An overnight worker obviously will go to bed in the morning.*

CHAPTER 9: Nature's 9 for the FAMILY: babies, kids and teens

PARENTS TO BE

Plan to give your baby the best start by getting healthy YOURSELVES first! I always tell people that you cannot make a good sandwich out of two moldy pieces of bread.☹ Keep in mind babies receive half of their DNA/genetic information from mom and half from dad. Therefore, if you both or even one of you is already sickly then you will pass that to the baby too! It is a fabulous idea for couples who want to have children to PREPARE their health for one year prior to "trying" to have a baby. They can be losing weight if necessary, taking vitamins, juicing and filling their bodies with nutrition while also detoxing their bodies with systematic cleansing and getting back in tune with Nature's 9. Mom can take herbs that help with breast milk production. Once they have completed the year they can offer the BEST genetic information to the baby. **I have had people-including doctors-laugh at me when I mention this, which makes me really MAD then SAD.** ☹☹

We spend a lot of time planning and preparing for other things in our lives such as buying a car. **Do we just say eenie—meenie—miney—moe to buy a house?** NO! We look at many houses: we analyze neighborhoods, how close is the house to work/schools and family; will the number of rooms in the house be enough; do we want a few levels or just one; is there a garage or street parking; will there be room for a garden or pets. We even begin saving money YEARS before so we can get the exact house we want. We haggle and negotiate over price and closing costs to get the best deal and live in the best area.

Why do we spend SO little time preparing for the greatest investment that we can create which is our children? Who benefits the most from the preparation? THE BABY! Did you know that some illnesses such as neural tube defects--birth defects of the brain and spinal cord--can be caused by a nutritional deficiency of the B vitamin Folic Acid! If the baby had had enough of this vitamin when their spine was developing then they would not be paralyzed in childhood and adulthood! Another neural tube defect prevents the baby's brain from developing! We cannot live without a brain and so usually, this will lead to a spontaneous abortion of the baby from mom's body before 9 months. Now, genetics may also cause neural tube defects but the point is to give your baby as much help AS YOU can control! You can control cleansing and taking vitamins so that when you decide to get pregnant the baby will already have what they need and get the best genetics! This is why getting into good shape and then doing the proper prenatal protocols is VERY important and will affect the ENTIRE lifetime of your child. YOU benefit too, since you can watch your child grow up healthily and happily instead of spending all of their time with doctors and hospitals! Of course we cannot control ALL illnesses just through preparation, since we know that "the universe" controls many aspects of life but I say at least TRY to prepare as much as possible.

I REPEAT: _BOTH_ MOM AND DAD MUST PREPARE. THERE IS NO POINT TO HAVE A SANDWICH WITH ONE NICE SLICE OF BREAD AND ONE GREEN MOLDY SLICE.☹

PARENTS to BE: Nutrition and supplements!

Both parents need to eat healthily so you can each pass a very nice "slice of bread" or DNA/Genetics to the baby when you do begin "trying" to get pregnant. See the nutrition section in chapter 8 and then do this as well:

- Minimum **50 grams of protein a day**—you can see a list of protein sources in chapter 11—we *need protein for EVERYTHING in body*
- **Little to NO unhealthy or bad food or sugar** *destroys the body*
- A good **multivitamin without iron**—we *need vitamins and minerals for basic function and to get healthy!* *If your iron levels are low then you may need a multivitamin with iron but check with your doctor first because having too much iron in the body can become toxic/harmful so we usually do not recommend people to take iron unless you are low. Get your iron in iron rich foods like dark leafy vegetables, beets/beet greens, beans, raisins and healthy red meats. *Red meats have highest and best forms of iron.*
- A good **probiotic**—*healthy bacteria for immune and digestion function!*
- **Vitamin D** drops—put under tongue—*needed in over 300 places in body!*
- A quality **fish oil/essential fatty acid/Omega 3s**—*helps build body!*
- **L-Glutamine**—*an amino acid that feeds healthy bacteria. Helps digestion!*

See chapter 17 "Dr. Megan's favorite supplements" section for my favorite supplement brands. Remember, you also need to follow the other eight of Nature's 9 so see chapter 8 for that information.

I AM PREGNANT: Nutrition and supplements!

Good job! ☺ Now *dads*, you still need to support mom! Do not think that you can eat junk now because mom does not need to see temptation foods in the house! Therefore dad if you want to eat badly, DO IT ALONE outside of the house and do not bring bad foods home or talk about eating bad foods! Pregnancy can be a time of true food cravings and it is usually for bad and unhealthy foods and mom needs to maintain a VERY healthy nutrition plan while pregnant and breast-feeding (if breast-feeding is possible). *Moms*, you are "eating for two" now so review the nutrition section in the Nat 9 and do these as well. There are a few changes:

- Minimum **<u>100</u> grams of protein a day**—*helps decrease developing high blood pressure with pregnancy*
- **Fiber**-*helps keep constipation away!* See chapter 11 for fiber sources.
- **Little to NO unhealthy or bad food or sugar** –*helps decrease developing diabetes with pregnancy*
- A good **multivitamin <u>WITH</u> iron** in a good form meaning a non-constipating iron form that is easy for the body to use like Iron Bis-Glycinate. *One multivitamin product is **Innate Response Formulas brand "Baby and Me Trimester I and II**. It may be necessary to supplement with

iron separately if the multivitamin does not have enough--*It is very common for mom to become anemic or have low red blood cells/semi-trucks with pregnancy and this is bad because then neither mom nor baby gets the supplies they need!*

- A good **probiotic**
- **Vitamin D** drops
- A quality **fish oil**
- **L-Glutamine**
- **Vitamin B6**—*you may need high doses of this for nausea*
- **Fresh Ginger root**—*can make tea for nausea and to help blood move better*

Note: In western medicine, it is generally not advisable to take ANY herbs within the first three months of pregnancy when the baby's development is the most sensitive. This would include taking supplements with herbs in them. It is best to wait until the middle to near end of the second trimester/months 5-6 before introducing herbs especially if you have never used the specific herb(s) before. It is also not advisable for you to take most herbs while breast-feeding. Please work with a knowledgeable health care professional if you want to use herbs in pregnancy and breast-feeding.

I believe that herbal warnings are exaggerated, especially since around the rest of the world, mothers are using herbs during pregnancy but I just thought that I would mention it anyway. Most medical literature confirms that Ginger and Chamomile are safe at any point throughout pregnancy. However, be sure to work with a health professional trained in the use of herbs during pregnancy.

Double Note: Most of the things that are really harming your baby NO ONE avoids: eating WAY TOO MUCH SUGAR, not drinking enough water and letting trash build up inside of your body, using caffeine (this is a drug!) and a bunch of other abuses! I have not even mentioned yet all the toxic medications that many women are using while pregnant! Ok. There. I just mentioned it. **So really, the baby's first drug dealer is mom.** ☹ **However, NO ONE restricts those bad things. OH NO. Just blame the herbs and supplements. ALWAYS.** ☹ True, there are some very strong herbs that absolutely can hurt the baby's development or even cause your baby hotel/uterus to send out the baby much too early but these herbs are not commonly used in supplements or found easily in health food stores. You have to really search for them. Anyway, I am finished yelling about how unfairly herbs are treated. I have had a little angry fit. ☹☹ But it is over now. Let us move on!

Remember: Have regular visits with your obstetrician/pregnancy doctor.

I AM PREGNANT: Exercise!

It is important for mom to be physically active as well. If you NEVER exercised before then light walking is usually fine for most women. Try to walk quickly for at least 15 minutes a day or minimum 3 days a week. If you were already very active before pregnancy (jogging, dancing etc.) then usually you can continue your activity to some degree. Consult with your obstetrician to make sure your level of activity can correspond with the months of pregnancy, the baby's position and any other health problems you or the baby may have.

Note: Just because you are pregnant does not mean you should lie around and not exercise! Many studies show that consistent physical activity helps labor! Women in poorer countries who spend most of their time walking everywhere and moving a lot during pregnancy tend to have very quick and easy births—labor can last 3-6 hours or less! They also have faster recovery time after birth than women in "rich" countries where physical activity is low!

Story: While I was in medical school, we had a banquet on the back lawn of the school. The organizers had invited a Capoeira group as part of the entertainment. Capoeira is a mix of African, Caribbean and South American dance as well as martial arts movements. It involves much jumping and kicking high into the air as well as twisting, turning and rolling along the ground. There was a woman in the group who was jumping high up, she did a twisting karate kick in the air and then landed in a squat--your knees are bent and your head and chest are close to your knees--and **she was EIGHT MONTHS PREGNANT!** While she was in the air, I wanted to run up to her with my arms outstretched and get underneath her to try to catch the baby in case it fell out when she landed! Anyway, even if the baby had popped out it probably would have just rolled across the lawn and then gotten up and started dancing with mama. ☺ She did the ENTIRE routine and was JUST as fast and active as the other women AND men in the group! I mean, I remember thinking "man, I cannot jump up three feet into the air and land into a squat! And I am not even pregnant with a watermelon belly"! That woman really was a rock star! ☺☺ This is not typical pregnant woman activity level. Please do not try this at home if you are pregnant. Do not try this even if you are <u>not</u> pregnant but just out of shape. ☹ The point is that she was clearly active before and during pregnancy.

I AM PREGNANT: Other therapies!
There are additional therapies that help mama "bear" and baby "cub" during pregnancy:

- **Mayan Abdominal Massage**—helps position baby and ease labor
- **Acupuncture**—helps mom and baby's organs and baby position
- **Chiropractic Adjustments**--helps baby and mom's organs and brain

It is great to have your newborn baby visit a chiropractor trained to work with newborns just after the birth (meaning in that same week of birth) so that they can have some of their bones and muscles realigned.
Although a vaginal birth is the natural and best way to have a birth, it is not easy for mom OR baby! Imagine if you had to squeeze through a very tight space headfirst.☹ A chiropractor can help baby's head bones, shoulders and spine get back where they should be and this will help baby's inside organs-heart, lungs etc. and muscles too! See chapter 19 under Dr. Megan's Georgia health professional referrals for some references!

BABY IS HERE!

VACCINATIONS: THE ESSENTIALS TO BE WELL INFORMED

Most of us do not relish the idea of getting a vaccine, whether in childhood or adulthood. However, the idea behind vaccination is good: expose the body to a small, controlled threat so that the body can prepare itself for any future, larger threat and kill the infectious bacteria/virus (organism). Vaccines are either **(1)** "live" meaning it is a living virus/ bacteria **(2)** "attenuated" meaning it is a less harmful part of a living virus/bacteria **(3)** "killed" if the organism is already dead. Some vaccines may contain harmful ingredients such as mercury, aluminum, formaldehyde or animal components that may provoke long-term ill effects in an individual. So how should one navigate the vaccination issue, whether in childhood for school or as an adult for work/recreational travel/preventative protection?

To vaccinate or not to vaccinate? That is the question!
The best way to decide if you or your child should be vaccinated--provided it is not mandatory for school or work--is to weigh:

(1) Risk of exposure high risk versus low risk
(2) Effects of the vaccine short-term versus long-term
(3) Effects of the disease or illness short-term versus long-term
(4) Health status of individual strong health versus weak health

For example, if a person has a low risk of exposure to the organism--and the resulting disease/illness it would cause is mild, then it may not be necessary to vaccinate. However, even if a person is at a low risk for catching the organism, but the disease/illness is <u>very severe or life threatening</u>--due to the individual's age or health status--then perhaps it is better to get that vaccine.

Additionally, there are some "homeopathic vaccines"/preparations for certain organisms. For any age group or health status, it is best to avoid taking multiple "live" vaccines.

Who is most at risk for catching an infectious organism?
Generally speaking, populations which are at risk for serious complications with certain viruses and bacteria are pregnant women, children under 2 years old, people with poor immune system function such as those with autoimmune diseases, HIV/AIDS or cancer, and the elderly.

Who should potentially avoid/limit certain vaccines?*
- Anyone who has had a serious bad reaction to the vaccine before--rashes, difficulty breathing etc.
- Anyone with cold/flu symptoms–*the body is already in a weakened state*
- Anyone with any other active infection elsewhere on/in the body
- Anyone with severe immune system deficiency-*those with Autoimmune diseases, Cancer, HIV/AIDS*
- Those with ANY diagnosed illness—seizures, heart or lung diseases etc.
- Those with Autistic Spectrum disease
- In pregnancy

Consult with your health care provider(s) to know which vaccines may be harmful for you/your child.

Transmission, Exposure Risk, Vaccine Side Effects, Disease Side Effects.
This section will give basic information about the most common vaccines. ***Childhood*** traditional vaccination schedules as well as a potential alternative schedule follow this section. For ***travel*** vaccines go to www.cdc.gov to see those recommended for the country/destination.

A few definitions first!
(1) Route of transmission means how you can get the virus/bacteria/organism. **Note:** this usually means by touching someone's blood or other body fluids, which are saliva/spit, urine/pee, or feces/poop. I know that you would not normally touch ANY of these on purpose but remember you are exposed to saliva/spit via kissing, drinking or eating from shared cups or utensils. You are exposed to pee, poop or blood if you touch door handles or any surfaces that someone else-who did not wash their hands well-has touched. All you need is to have a tiny cut in your skin that you are unaware of and the microorganism can crawl into the United States of You from there!☹

Medical procedures can also put you at risk for getting an infectious organism. Additionally you can get infectious microorganisms from your skin touching certain objects such as stepping on a nail, scraping your skin on a fence or coming in contact with dirt that has these microorganisms in them. If someone coughs or sneezes air droplets will often hang in the air for a few minutes before they drop down and you can walk by and breathe them in.☹ You can catch organisms by contact with animals and their poop, pee or spit. Lastly, insects that bite (mosquitoes, ticks, fleas) can also infect you with an organism when they pierce your skin. With so many ways for you to catch these microorganisms, aren't you glad that you have an immune system/internal police!

 Oh, by the way, **infectious** just means it can make you develop an infection or illness. It usually refers to a certain **microorganism**, which is a very small, usually mean, living thing that we cannot see with the naked eye—so we need a microscope. Common microorganisms are viruses, bacteria, fungi, and protozoans (parasites). I also may refer to microorganisms as **"bugs" or "bad bugs"**.

Elderly is someone older than 65 years old. An **infant** is a baby under 12 months old. I may forget and just type "baby" though. But you get the idea.

A person who is **"immune compromised"** has a serious illness that directly affects the immune system such as HIV/AIDS, Cancer or Autoimmune diseases like Lupus.

Some abbreviations: "mo" means months and "yo" means years old.

In the vaccine reaction section "typical" means the bad effects people most commonly get with the vaccine and "severe" means less common but more serious reactions that a person could get.

(2) Exposure risk means who is most likely to get the organism
(3) Vaccine side effects means the bad reactions you could have after you get the vaccine
(4) Disease side effects are the health problems you can develop if you <u>do not get the vaccine</u> and you catch the "bug" which then causes a disease or illness

An **illness** is short-term. Like a cold or flu, it makes you sick for a while but it does not last forever. A **disease** will make you sick for a very long time. Sometimes you can get an illness first that then makes you develop a disease. Example: if a bacteria messes up Pancreas city→Diabetes. Sometimes I use disease/illness interchangeably.

BOOK ALERT: Woo Hoo! Half way through the book!

Does anyone remember that Bon Jovi song? ♪Ohhhh, we're half way there, Oh

OH, living on a prayer♪...Ok enough singing, now let us keep learning. ☺

Hepatitis B Virus (Hep B)
- **Route of Transmission**: blood and body fluids, sexual intercourse
- **Highest exposure risk**: medical professionals; babies born vaginally to an infected mother; blood transfusion
- **Vaccine Side Effects**: **Typical**: flu-like; **Severe:** Autoimmune disease-body's immune system is confused and attacks itself (organs/muscles etc.) as well as infectious organisms; Nervous system problems; Guillain-Barré Syndrome (nerve disease-potentially lethal! ☹)
- **Disease Effects**: Liver dysfunction/chronic infection; Liver cancer

Rotavirus (RV)—one of the main viruses that cause the common cold
- **Route of Transmission**: person to person (unclean hands/poor hygiene);
- **Highest exposure risk:** every one by age 3
- **Vaccine Side Effects: Typical**: flu-like; **Severe:** Intussusception (intestinal folding)-rare
- **Disease Effects:** watery diarrhea--especially in kids less than 2yo→dehydration/too low water in body, vomiting, fever

Diptheria, Tetanus, Pertussis (DTP or DTaP)
- **Route of Transmission**: person to person/poor hygiene, contaminated surfaces (Diphtheria); puncture wound (Tetanus)-can be a puncture from an animal bite or a nail or object; respiratory/cough (Diphtheria, Pertussis)-*Adults can often be pertussis carriers and infect babies* ☹
- **Highest exposure risk**: travel-particularly to Russia (Diphtheria-rare in US); rusty nails (Tetanus); less than 6 mo old can require hospitalization, less than 3 mo old can be lethal/kill! ☹(Pertussis)
- **Vaccine Side Effects**: **Typical**: redness at injection site, swelling, fever; **Severe**: nervous system dysfunction, may worsen asthma
- **Disease Effects**: Diptheria (sore throat, fever, difficulty swallowing due to a thin membrane that forms in the throat-potentially lethal! ☹); Tetanus (lockjaw); Pertussis (whooping cough)

Haemophilus Influenza type b (Hib)
- **Route of Transmission**: respiratory/cough
- **Highest exposure risk**: everyone but disease effects are more severe in those less than 2 yo
- **Vaccine Side Effects: Typical**: flu-like; *vaccine not recommended for more than 5 yo*
- **Disease Effects**. Meningitis is swelling of the brain layers potentially lethal! ☹-meningitis symptoms are fever, stiff neck, vomiting, confusion, lethargy, irritability, seizures; Epiglottitis (swelling of the epiglottis in throat-potentially lethal! ☹); Pneumonia

Pneumococcus (PCV)
- **Route of Transmission**: person to person/poor hygiene; respiratory/cough
- **Highest exposure risk**: infants, elderly. With vaccine rare beyond 2 yo though now can be exposed via different strains.
- **Vaccine Side Effects: Typical**: flu-like; **Severe**: seizures (rare 1:20,000) *if given with Hib, Pertussis or Polio may lower efficacy of those vaccines. Those with a soy allergy may have a significant adverse reaction.*
- **Disease Effects**: Pneumonia; Sepsis (bacterial infection of the blood-potentially lethal!☹)--especially elderly; Meningitis-especially elderly (higher fatality/kill rate in both infants and elderly than Hib)

Inactivated Polio Virus (IPV)

- **Route of Transmission:** person to person/poor hygiene; bats and skunks
- **Highest exposure risk:** eliminated in western hemisphere; travel to sub-Saharan Africa, India; non-vaccinated people.
- **Vaccine Side Effects: Typical:** local skin allergic reaction; **Severe:** difficulty breathing, palpitations/very strong heart beats
- **Disease Effects:** initially flu-like; Meningitis; progressive muscle weakness, paralysis of limbs; with SV-40 virus species brain tumors and bone cancers (research done in monkey cells shows this effect)

Measles, Mumps and Rubella Virus (MMR)

- **Route of Transmission:** respiratory/saliva; direct touch/contact with rash pus/fluid
- **Highest exposure risk:** rare in U.S. (especially measles)
- **Vaccine Side Effects: Typical:** fever, dizziness; **Severe:** fainting, poor balance, seizure, joint pain, ear infection; *with Tylenol use may contribute to Autistic disorder*
- **Disease Effects:** diarrhea, rash (Measles); Parotitis-swelling of salivary glands in neck; Orchitis-swelling of the testes in males-more post puberty; may be related to attack on pancreas→Diabetes (Mumps); Encephalitis-inflammation of parts of the brain-potentially lethal! ☹; Juvenile Arthritis; joint pain–especially adult females (Rubella)

Hepatitis A Virus (Hep A)

- **Route of Transmission:** person to person/poor hygiene; contaminated surfaces
- **Highest exposure risk:** 5-14 yo; more prevalent in western portion of US but really anyone
- **Vaccine Side Effects: Typical:** fatigue, fever, headache; **Severe:** may decrease efficacy of pertussis vaccine; may provoke seizures in less than 2 yo; may want to avoid in those with liver disease.
- **Disease Effects:** RARE; liver dysfunction (mild); jaundice-especially in children less than 6 yo. Jaundice can happen when Bile--juice from the liver--builds up around the body. It can turn the white part of your eyes and nails a yellow green color. If you have fair skin, it can make you look a little green too. ☹

Influenza (Flu) Virus
- **Route of Transmission**: person to person/poor hygiene, respiratory/cough
- **Highest exposure risk**: mostly elderly; infants;
- **Vaccine Side Effects**: **Typical**: fever, fatigue, arthritis; **Severe:** Guillain- Barré Syndrome; potentially lung symptoms; may cause fetal harm if administered in pregnancy; may worsen asthma.
- **Disease Effects**: flu; hospitalization and/or death. Mainly in elderly. From 1990 to 1999 more than 90% of deaths in elderly! ☹

Varicella Virus
- **Route of Transmission**: person to person,
- **Highest exposure risk**: Chicken Pox is a common childhood disease-more severe in an adult who never had the disease as a child
- **Vaccine Side Effects**: **Typical**: rash; flu-like; **Severe:** Guillain-Barré Syndrome; Shingles; Varicella breakthrough increased by 2.5 times if given less than 30 days following MMR vaccine.
- **Disease Effects**: Chicken Pox (Varicella); Shingles (Herpes Zoster)-may recur after a previous infection with Chicken Pox--typically in adulthood and is more severe than Chicken Pox.

Meningococcal (MCV)
- **Route of Transmission**: person to person,
- **Highest exposure risk**: military barracks, schools; especially infants less than 1 yo; those with immune dysfunction diseases
- **Vaccine Side Effects**: **Typical**: rash; flu-like; **Severe:** fainting spells, jerking movements-happens more in adolescents, very bad allergic reactions.
- **Disease Effects**: Meningitis

Tuberculosis (BCG)
- **Route of Transmission**: person to person/touch; respiratory/cough
- **Highest exposure risk**: medical professionals; airplane travel
- **Vaccine Side Effects**: **Typical**: local injection soreness; **Severe:** lung disease
- **Disease Effects**: severe cough; potentially fatal in the immune compromised.

Human Papilloma Virus (HPV)
- **Route of Transmission**: sexual contact/intercourse
- **Highest exposure risk**: teens or early 20's; anyone using non-latex condoms*
- **Vaccine Side Effects**: **Typical**: headache, fatigue **Severe:** bad allergic reaction
- **Disease Effects**: *women*-cervical cancer; *anyone*-genital warts→anal cancer

*Viruses are small enough to pass through non-latex or natural condoms. ☹

CHILD HOOD VACCINATIONS

In 1974 there were only 14 vaccinations recommended from birth to 6 years old. In 2009 there were 34 vaccinations recommended through 6 years of age. Vaccinations begin at birth, but a baby's immune system is very basic and truly does not begin to form until approximately after 6 months old. In a vaginal birth, the baby can access some of its mother's immune cells/bacteria as it is passing through the birth canal. Additionally, through breast feeding the child can obtain antibodies--little "flags" that are put onto bad "bugs" like viruses/bacteria--that signal immune/police cells to destroy them. Otherwise, the baby is really using mom's immune system. Therefore vaccinating a child with multiple types of organisms before it even has an immune system that truly operates may not be of the best benefit. The vaccines are given during these age ranges.

TRADITIONAL CHILDHOOD VACCINE SCHEDULE Birth--12 years (www.CDC.gov)

Hepatitis (HepB)--Birth--2 mo, 6--18 mo
Rotavirus (RV)---2, 4, 6 mo
Diptheria, Tetanus, Pertussis (DTaP)----------------------2, 4, 6, 15-18, 4-6yo, 11-12 yo*
Haemophilus Influenzae type B (Hib)--------------------2, 4, 6, 12--15 mo
Pneumococcal (PCV)--------------------------------------2, 4, 6, 12--15 mo
Inactivated Polio (IPV)------------------------------------2, 4, 6--18 mo , 4-6 yo
Influenza/Flu--Yearly
Measles, Mumps, Rubella (MMR)------------------------12--15 mo, 4-6 yo
Varicella--12, 15 mo, 4-6 yo
Hepatitis A (Hep A)---12--23 mo
Meningococcal (MCV)--------------------------------------11--12 yo
Humanpapilloma (HPV)------------------------------------11-12 yo

*They recommend Tdap at 11-12 yo only if the child missed the DTap earlier

POTENTIAL ALTERNATIVE VACCINE SCHEDULE

Again, understanding newborn/infants limited immune development it may be wise to space out vaccinations. Discuss this with your pediatrician and alternative healthcare provider.

- 2 mo—PCV
- 3 mo---Hib
- 4 mo---DTaP
- 6 mo---PCV
- 8 mo---DTaP
- 10 mo---Hib
- 12 mo---DTaP

- 15 mo---PCV
- 18 mo---Hib
- 20 mo—Dtap
- 8-12 yo-MMR; Varicella (before puberty-more than 30 days away from MMR); Hep B (before puberty)

WOW! THIS IS A LOT OF INFORMATION! A LITTLE HELP PLEASE?

The Hepatitis B vaccine is given much too early, in my opinion. Unless the mother has Hepatitis, AND the baby is born via vaginal birth, then the baby has little to no likelihood of catching Hepatitis B. Remember, many babies do not even begin to develop their immune system/police until around 6 months old so before that they are using mom's antibodies/post-its or "mug shots". **Analogy:** *Giving a baby with no immune system/police certain vaccines is like bringing in a bus of prisoners/criminals into a neighborhood where there is no police station and releasing the criminals to run around freely.*

They give most vaccines in a certain schedule because it is more convenient for the medical system and for the parents to get many vaccines at once instead of having the parents return more frequently with the child. However, this schedule does not benefit the health of the child.

It is true that there are **certain vaccines that may be important** to get very early in the baby's life simply because the disease could kill the baby and that is much worse than the vaccine's bad effects. Examples would be Pneumococcus (PCV) and Haemophilus Influenzae (Hib).

Human papillomavirus (HPV) has many strains/types that can make you sick. The vaccine usually only uses the two most common types. Abstinence during high-risk ages is best; and or latex condom use 100% of the time; low sexual partner numbers.

Other vaccines such as the Influenza/flu vaccine are **largely useless** for most people whether a baby or an adult. The flu virus mutates/changes disguises so rapidly and so often that we are only guessing which disguise the virus might be wearing at any given time. Then based upon our guesses we attempt to make a vaccine to kill the virus. **You can _still_ get sick after having vaccines!** *Analogy: a bulletproof vest only protects your chest. Not your head, arms, or legs! You can still be shot elsewhere! You have to protect/strengthen the ENTIRE body.* It is more important to focus on keeping the United States of You healthy by doing Nature's 9 and if the flu or whatever virus/bacteria does invade your body then your immune system/police will kill it!

VACCINE RESOURCES
Websites: www.ThinkTwice.com and www.holisticmoms.org
Books: Make An Informed Vaccine Decision[75] and Childhood Vaccination[76].

Recall that if you or your child must get a traditional vaccine because of your work or their school and you **cannot** escape it, then just help your/their body deal with the vaccine before and after by using water, healthy diet, probiotics, Vitamin C and Vitamin D. There is no need for you to be fired from your job--which makes you lose your home and then you must live under a bridge--all because you refused to get a vaccine! It is not that serious. Avoid living under bridges. ☹

*Thank you to **Dr. Matthew Baral**[54] for the literature insights!*

FOOD INTRODUCTION FOR BABIES 0-2 years old.
One you do have your baby then this is a good schedule to introduce foods to baby's system. The way that we introduce food into a baby's system can affect their health right now and years ahead!

- **Best to keep breast feeding as long as possible**—only mom's milk minimum 4-6 months then adding in foods along with mom's milk. One year of breast feeding is optimal and many naturopathic doctors suggest even up until 2 years old—of course by then baby has teeth so if they try to chew the boob you are in trouble.☹ *Mom's milk is full of antibodies and nutrition!* There are **lactation/breast feeding coaches** to help you breast feed if you are having a hard time. If after using a lactation specialist you are still unable to breast feed because of pain, the baby will not latch on or perhaps you do not produce enough milk then you may have to use formula. Use formulas that are partially or extensively hydrolyzed-meaning they break apart the formula using water, which makes it easier for baby to digest. **Avoid cow's milk and soy formulas** because they are highly allergenic foods meaning they will cause baby to have bad reactions to it-so try to get formulas from goat's milk instead. There are also homemade formulas that you can make. Look for a naturopathic pediatrician to help you with this. **NOTE:** *remember when you are breast feeding you are still "eating for two" so **MOM needs to still avoid highly allergenic foods as much as possible!** These are: Dairy (anything from a cow), Eggs, Wheat, Peanuts, Soy, Corn, Citrus and Fish. Yes, I know those are many things to avoid, but this is all in an effort to help the BABY, **who did not ask to be born**! **You owe it to them**! So give the baby a hand and help them have a good start! It is only for a few months so no whining or complaining here please!* ☺

- **Best to make your own baby food if possible**; or look for baby foods that are certified USDA organic. At minimum, pick foods that do not have SUGAR or any other additives, fillers or colors since *these will decrease baby's heart, digestive and immune system functions.*

- **Can introduce solid foods, lightly and continuing with mom's milk** between 6-8 mo, or when it is apparent that baby can tolerate them AVOIDING ALL foods that are **highly allergenic: WHEAT, SOY, DAIRY, EGGS, OATMEAL, CORN, PEANUTS, CITRUS and FISH** until at least 12-18 mo then you can add them in twice a week. Add in allergenic foods one at a time (meaning do not have corn and eggs in the same meal) and look for **food reactions:** rashes, fever, earaches, or baby is burping more. Pooping changes: pooping more or less, poop has major color change, poop has a major change in odor like it has a stronger smell or has strange smells like "fruity". Other signs of Baby Digestion city problems: baby cries more/fussier, begins sleeping a lot more or a lot less than usual or frequent colds, flus or cough/runny nose or gooky eye mucus (gooky is not a medical term ☺). *Early introduction of allergenic foods into the diet can lead to food sensitivities, digestive troubles and autoimmune illnesses in childhood or even well into adulthood.*

  ➢ **6-8 mo**: emphasis on GREEN VEGETABLES and some fruits. We want foods with high iron content that will help the heart and circulation as well as the system as a whole. *High iron foods* are: swiss chard, dulse, mustard greens, leeks, apricots, kale, pumpkin seed, spinach, broccoli, pumpkin, peas. *Medium iron foods*: collard greens, beets, figs, raisins, prunes, endive, green beans, parsley, kelp, leaf lettuce, blueberries, banana, raspberry, blackberries, applesauce, sprouts, Jerusalem artichokes.

  ➢ **9-12 mo**: can add in proteins in the form of beans: lima, kidney, black, navy, pinto and all other types of beans.

  ➢ **12-15 mo**: can add in proteins in meat forms: poultry and lamb. Goat sources are less allergenic and more nutritious than cow/bovine. Avoid pork and shellfish.

  ➢ 12-15 mo: can add in grains like rice, amaranth, quinoa

  ➢ **15-18 mo**: can add in oatmeal

  ➢ **18-24 mo**: can add in products containing wheat.

BABY RESOURCES

- Book: **Infant Nutrition** by Dr. Mark Percival-chiropractor and naturopathic doctor/ND-which discusses how to prepare food and get the maximum nutrition out of food.
- Book: **Encyclopedia of Natural Healing for Children and Infants** by Dr. Mary Bove, ND.
- Book: **Conceiving Healthy Babies**: An herbal guide to support preconception, pregnancy and lactation by Dawn Combs.
- Book: **The Natural Pregnancy Book** by Dr. Aviva Jill Romm, MD and Ina May Gaskin.
- **Organics Happy Family**[46]. Foods for mama, baby and toddlers.
- **Baby bullet** appliance: the baby version of the "magic bullet" can assist with food preparation.

WOMEN'S RESOURCES

- Book: **Women's Encyclopedia of Natural Medicine** by Dr. Tori Hudson, ND. Discusses ALL things woman!
- Book: **Botanical Medicines for Women's Health** by Dr. Aviva Romm, MD.

MEN'S RESOURCES

I have yet to find a book that I like dedicated to ALL aspects of men's health. Usually the books just focus on the prostate. They do not address other male issues such as erectile difficulties, fitness, aging, hormones and just how much you men hate doctors and NEVER go until you are crawling on the floor or until your spouse/partner has harassed you to death.☹ I will keep on looking though.
If someone hears of one please let me know.☺ Anyway, you can use the information in my book for everything else and use one of these books for when you are trying to heal your prostate specifically.

- Book: **The Natural Way to A Healthy Prostate** by Dr. Michael B. Schachter, MD.
- Book: **Natural Prostate Healers: A breakthrough Program for Preventing and Treating Common Prostate Problems Without Drugs or Surgery** by Mike Fillon.

MY FAVORITE BASIC SUPPLEMENTS FOR KIDS

Kids are growing and so they really need basic nutrients to help their little bodies develop! Many of the supplements that you can just buy off the shelves at random stores are not good quality so it is not wise to waste money there. Read more about supplements in chapter 17. Here are my favorites right now:

- **MULTIVITAMIN**—Perque brand Lifeguard Chewables (perkies) cherry/raspberry flavor—*vitamins and minerals are for energy and basic function!*
- **FISH OIL**--Barleans brand Kids Omega Swirl-you can dose based on their weight--*fish oils are essential for building the body organ and parts.*
- **PROBIOTIC**—Klaire Labs brand Ther-Biotic Infant formula (0-2 years)* Pharmax brand HLC Child (2 years to 6 years) and then Genestra brand HMF Child (7 years to 12 years)-- *probiotics assist in digestion and immune system function and are essential in maintaining a strong system.*

*Note: babies and children less than 2 years old can also take probiotics but you need to work with a qualified health professional when dosing that.

NATURE'S 9 FOR BABIES KIDS AND TEENS!

AIR #1 for kids
- **Jail time**—colds, flus and allergies
- **Avoid Jail!**—take babies outside and sit in the sun with them. Kids and teens should have mandatory time outside daily especially since many schools have removed physical exercise and or outside time; meaning NO spending hours inside playing video games or TV right after school.
- **How to do it**—have them play games outside, you can play too! Old games are still fun: hop scotch, tag, kickball, throwing a baseball.

WATER #2 for kids
- **Jail time**—constipation, being sleepy in school, fainting at sports practices
- **Avoid Jail!** —drink plenty! For kids and teens half their body weight in ounces.
- **How to do it**—make it a game! When my two oldest nephews J and P were little we used to "race" and see who could finish their glass of water first! They would always win. ☹ Of course their glasses were MUCH smaller than mine. I also have "races" with my other nephew A now!

BONUS: NATURAL "SPORTS DRINK" RECIPE

Kids and teens that play sports sweat a lot and we lose water AND salt when we sweat. You do not believe me? Next time you are sweating lick some part of your body and you will see it tastes salty! Pick a nice spot like right below your lip...not somewhere gross like your underarm.☹ To take salt back into the body with water we ALSO need a little sugar. This is why companies have created sports drinks to help put some of the minerals back in your body. However, most sports drinks have too much sugar, which is NEVER good for the body. Here is a natural recipe that is healthier. You can use it during and after sports as well as other times of heavy sweating like while doing yardwork...another thing I hate ☹ but I still hate cooking more.☹☹

- 2 cups of water (remember one cup is 8 ounces or 250mL)
- 1/2 cup of any type fruit juice (no added sugar)
- 1/8 teaspoon of salt (sea salt preferred)

Shake it well and drink!

Note: remember, NO cold drinks of ANY kind while kids (or adults) are sick! I mean do not drink any drink directly from the refrigerator or put ice cubes in drinks. At a restaurant, even some drinks without ice are still very cold. Avoid drinks colder than room temperature when sick. Takes body energy to warm up a cold drink.

NUTRITION #3 for kids

It is VERY important to teach babies and kids healthy nutrition from the very beginning of their lives and onward! YOU ARE WHAT YOU EAT! How can you expect them to grow well if they are eating rubbish?
Remember ANYTHING you put in their mouths is either helping or hurting them!
Try to make most of what they eat HELP them!

- **Jail time**—rashes, earaches, stomachaches, asthma, poor concentration in school, overweight or obese kids.
- **Avoid Jail!—Babies:** follow the principles for food introduction above. **Kids:** teach them about healthy foods! Practice what you preach! Do not buy junk or unhealthy food for the house. Do not have sugary foods, drinks or candy in the house.

- **How to do it**—my formula W2H2 and the basic nutrition rules still apply to them. Kids LOVE to learn so go on the internet together and look up why green vegetables are good. Have a mini-garden in your home! Use one little pot and grow a tomato or an herb! It will be a fun way to spend time together learning about food and appreciating mother Earth! Plan a field trip to a local farm or library to learn about food there!

SLEEP #4 for kids
This is SUPER important for babies, kids and teens! Sleep is a time for the body to rest and build. Have you ever wondered why babies SLEEP all day for the first few months of life? They should not be tired since they really have not been doing anything while they were inside mom's belly! They are not TIRED! Sleep is a MAJOR way for the body to BUILD new things and FIX or RECYCLE broken things! Therefore, since a baby is building a body to last for a lifetime, it must sleep for the first few months! This is why as we age we need less and less sleep because we spend more time maintaining what we already have versus building. This area is really abused when you let your kids stay up late watching TV or playing. I know it is hard to control what teens do because you yourself go to bed and they may decide to stay up so I am speaking more about kids 2 years old to 12 years old. I once had a parent come to the clinic complaining about their 4 year old's performance at school and then they told me that they let the kid stay up with them until 11pm at night!

- **Jail time**--poor performance at school, temper tantrums.
- **Avoid Jail!**—kids 2 years-12 years aim for 10-12 hours of sleep so bedtime no later than 730pm-8pm. Teens need about 8-10 hours.
- **How to do it**--sleep routine *one hour before bedtime* still applies. For younger kids you can play a sleepy time song for them and maybe read or tell them a story--yes, the old things still work! No scary stories. ☹
  For teens you may have to confiscate electronics like tablets, computers, cell phones, video games or the remote controls/power cords for these things and return them in the morning, if you see that they persistently do not go to bed on time. YES, you can do this; *you have the right and the duty* to look out for their well-being! YOU are the one paying for these devices-and doctor visits-if they do not take care of themselves anyway!

EXERCISE #5 for kids

Many things have contributed to childhood obesity in this country and of course poor nutrition is #1 but the next factors would be the lack of exercise and the boom in electronics. Kids are fatter than their parents are and begin gaining weight at a much younger age.

- **Jail time--**high blood pressure, low self-esteem, low quality of life.
- **Avoid Jail!**—do not let kids and teens come home from school and just sit on the couch. Have mandatory exercise time. Outside exercise is best then they can get fresh air, sunshine and movement (3 of Nat's 9) all at one time!
- **How to do it**—Aerobic is best*—meaning where your heart is pumping fast and you are sweating! Do games! Give **kids 2 years to 6 years old** a head start to run in one direction while you count down aloud and then your run after them! **Kids 6-10 years old** you can have a jumping contest and jump up and down in place and see who wins! Blob tag is super fun! In blob tag one person is "it" and they have to try to chase a second person and tag them. Then the first person and the second hold hands and run after other people—each of the first two "it" people can tag a person with their free hand. As people are tagged, they also have to join hands with the original first two. It gets harder and harder to avoid being tagged when you are in a confined area with a big "blob" chasing you! Jumping ropes and Hula Hoops are still fun at this age too! **Kids 10 and up** you can use video game consoles that have exercise games. For example, once when my 3 nephews J, P and A were all visiting, we played the dancing game on the Wii! I do not like video games but I had a lot of fun picking my favorite songs and following the dance moves! Plus, I was sweating like a horse after only a few minutes! Electronics are not all bad. ☺ Do not forget you can use YouTube/Internet for exercise too. Try to get at least 20-30 minutes a day.

GROUNDING: TIME OUT IN NATURE #6 for kids
Gone are the summer days when kids would leave home in the morning and spend the entire day outside riding bikes, playing games, climbing trees, swimming in lakes or playing in a puddle. Kids today spend MOST of their time inside.

- **Jail time--**frequent colds/flus, sinus infections, low focus
- **Avoid Jail!**—take the kids to the park, back yard or wherever you see a patch of grass and just lie down on it. Roll over onto your stomach and look for bugs and signs of life! I was sitting outside the other day and I was excited to see the "helicopter" bugs! The ones with big wings and a very long thin body. After that I saw a humming bird and a praying mantis! Nature is fun to watch so get outside!

POSITIVE MINDSET/SPIRITUALITY #7 for kids
It is very sad to see a 70 year old person sitting in front of you and crying as they tell you about something mean their father, mother or caregiver said about them when they were 8 years old. ☹ Negative words and expressions are SO damaging to a kid, even 40, 50 and 60 years later! As a parent or guardian of a child, you must remember that the most important years in a child's life are from birth to about 7 years old! That is when they learn from YOU what it means to be a good versus a bad person, their role in life as a girl or boy, and how relationships work between a couple. They also form opinions about body image and develop mental and emotional stability. You may think that kids' and teens' friends are the most important factor to them, but studies show time and time again that PARENTS have the greatest impact on their children. More than their peers! Therefore, if you speak negatively to them (or about yourself) with regard to intelligence, body image, usefulness around the house or what they will be in life, they will BELIEVE it! Even years later it is difficult to undo the harm of a parent or guardian who has told a child that they are dumb, ugly, lazy, will never amount to much, and that they were a mistake. The children will believe your negative words and become all of those things or almost KILL themselves trying to prove you wrong and to be good enough in your eyes and the world's eyes! ☹

- **Jail time**--mental illness, acting out at school or home, gangs or affiliations where they can "belong", eating disorders, and self-mutilation.
- **Avoid Jail!**—Be sure to speak openly and honestly to your kids and teach them the lessons they need to learn but do it with positive reinforcement rather than with negative or demeaning words. Also if you acknowledge that there is a higher power in the universe, whomever or whatever you believe that higher power to be, that can also help a child cope better with their life image.
- **How to do it—Examples (1)** NEVER compare a child to their brother/sister or other person! "Why can't you be more like your brother who gets better grades/plays sports?" This only hurts the child and will foster sibling rivalry. Praise them for their good qualities. Help them work on weak ones. Everyone is unique! **(2)** Do not tell a child that THEY are bad, but instead that a certain BEHAVIOR is bad or harmful and explain why it can hurt them as well as others. **(3)** Calling them mean names like "fat" to motivate them to lose weight is not helpful, even if your intention is good because you want them to get healthy. Instead, tell them that they are overweight right now, but they can change that with the lifestyle choices they make. Girls are very susceptible to body image problems, particularly Whites and Asians who typically want to be very thin compared to Blacks and Latinas. Therefore, if a fair-skinned girl sees her mother figure *obsessing* about weight she will also start worrying about weight at a very young age. It is possible for doctors to see girls as young as 5 and 7 years old dieting in order to be thin! **(4)** Be sure to use positive words to encourage your kids: "You are smart, loved and I am proud of you, you are great". Nothing positive can come from being negative! Tell them once a week minimum!

PURPOSE #8 for kids

Kids really need to understand that their life has a purpose very early on. When you let them know that they are here to become a nice productive human being and to help other people as they help themselves, then they will be happier! When young people have nothing to work towards, they usually get very lazy and get into trouble!

- **Jail time**—drugs, alcohol, depression, thrill seeking behaviors.
- **Avoid Jail!**—Save the environment organizations, community events like gardens etc. Adopt-a-grandparent! Use the Internet and public libraries!
- **How to do this**--from very early on take kids to see different professionals: firemen, engineers, policemen, doctors, teachers, mechanics and more! Let them talk to these people and follow them around for a minute.

Ask kids what they want to be when they "grow up". This question stimulates them to think about their future. Buy kids **2 years old to 12 years old** toys in the profession that they like. **Example:** I used to know a little girl who wanted to be a doctor, so when I would see her, I would take over my stethoscope and other equipment and let her listen to my heart and lungs. A few times, she pronounced me "dead"! ☺ Look over the kids' homework with them even if you do not have a clue what the homework means.☺ It lets them know you care about the work they are doing. The idea is to motivate and encourage them to ASPIRE to be and do something with their lives! Higher learning is not for everyone and that is ok! Encourage them to get into a trade. For **13 years old and older,** they can get into activities such as feeding the homeless, helping clean up disaster areas or the highways, and even travel locally, nationally or internationally to build schools and communities! Let them visit children's hospitals and cheer up the kids there. Just remind them that there is more to life than what is going on in their little circle and to try to look out for fellow mankind and make someone's day brighter.☺

FUN! JUST FOR ME! #9 for kids

Kids usually have NO problem having fun. The idea here is to try to incorporate more family fun instead of just sending them out with friends or letting electronics take over the household.

- **Jail time--**irritability, poor focus. Loneliness.
- **Avoid Jail!—**turn your house into the "cool" house!
- **How to do it--**Have game night! For **little kids** you can do treasure hunts around the house with hidden clues and little fun things to find. For **older kids** you can do board games, and card games. Have a movie night with popcorn and everything! Let them invite friends! Again, it may seem lame to you and the kids may protest initially but they usually always enjoy themselves and then look forward to the time together. Kids really just want the adults in their lives to interact with them and ANY activity can be fun. **Story:** I was doing a house call once, and I was showing the individual how to make a certain tea, and a kid left his toys and electronics to watch me grate ginger! He had never seen a grater and he thought it was the coolest thing! I let him play with it a little bit. Even that turned into a game! Kids these days interact so much with electronics. However, nothing can substitute for human time and touch! The basic things are still fun to them! Remember that public libraries often have free events like puppet shows and free tickets to the zoo and other fun attractions for the family!

LAST ADVICE FOR PARENTS

You want your kids to be mentally, emotionally and physically strong right? Therefore, it is important to help them as much as you can. I have two main pieces of advice:

#1 You are a parent first, friend later—this means that it is important to instill discipline from a VERY early age, even by 6 months of age a baby should understand that if you say "no" you mean it. Do not be wishy-washy and say one thing but then do not follow through. Kids LOVE discipline and routine. They feel stable and know what to expect from you. Why? Because **as humans we are creatures of habit and love routine** or to know what to expect. *Analogy: Have you ever sat down on a chair with one bad chair leg? Sometimes the chair holds you, but it is shaking. Other times the chair does not hold you and it breaks and you fall to the floor! So half of the time you do not know if you should sit or not! You have to test the chair by putting only half your bum on it at a time! And if you do sit down you do not feel secure. Very annoying!* ☹

Your children feel this way when you are not consistent with what you say and do. Your "no" is really "yes"; your "go left" is actually "go right" and your "up" might be "down!" No wonder they are confused and simply decide to do whatever THEY want to do! **Establish yourself as the head of the house!** You make AND enforce the rules! If they break a rule then there are consequences. Follow through with discipline! Oh yes, they may be mad at you in the moment and try to put up a fight. Again **as humans, we try to resist change once we are used to something** being a certain way. However, many studies show that kids with a home routine and discipline (firm and loving parenting) are MUCH happier and healthier than kids whom the parents allow to do whatever they want to, whenever they want to. Do not be a shaky chair. ☹ Do not be a chair that is <u>too hard</u> either. ☹

In a two parent household be sure to NEVER fight in front of kids *especially* if it concerns the child in some way—what they should eat or how to discipline them. Both parents should agree. If you do argue in front of kids, you will always lose! Kids are SUPER smart and know how to play one parent against the other. In my home, I never even saw my parents argue until I was 17 years old! Either they agreed with each other right away or if they did not quite agree, they would tell us kids that they would talk about it and then get back with us about the decision. If they found out that I had tried to get around something that one parent told me by going to the other parent for permission (such as going behind mom's back after she told me "no" to ask permission from dad because he did not know that mom had already told me "no") then I was in **_BIG_** trouble.

I have seen parents in the office that argue in front of the child: one parent is "good cop" and the other is "bad cop" meaning one parent lets the child do everything and the other parent only disciplines. Kids need balance! Additionally, this kind of behavior will place a strain on the parents' relationship because one parent will always feel as if the other parent does not support them. In a two-parent household you must seriously work on this.

- **Set a routine (meal times, exercise, outside time, bedtime) AND establish house rules (about chores, fighting, bad language, curfews etc.)** and have age appropriate consequences for when the rules are broken. Very young children 6 months to about 4 years old generally do not have reasoning skills so it may be difficult to explain things to them. **Story:** *When my oldest nephew J was about one year old, he was in my room with me while I was styling my hair. He kept reaching for the curling iron and I had told him at least 4 times not to touch it because it was hot. I turned my back for a second and when I turned back around, he was reaching to pull the curling iron down. I decided to show him what "hot" meant. I took his tiny finger and placed it on the curling iron for not even half a second, he did not burn, but it was just long enough for him to feel the heat a little bit. Of course, he began to cry and at that time, I repeated for him not to touch the curling iron because it was hot. He only cried for a few seconds and then after that whenever he looked at the curling iron I could hear him saying "hot" "hot" and he was giving the curling iron mean looks and he did not try to touch it again.* ☺ Now I know some of you may think that was incorrect but I did that to **PROTECT him**. Babies and young kids up to 4 years old cannot reason well and generally do not understand explanations because they have not yet lived the experience. I had already told him MANY times it would hurt him. **Babies and young kids need to learn OBEDIENCE first:** that they need to listen to you when you speak and obey you the FIRST time you say something and that if they do not, there is a painful consequence. Therefore, age appropriate corporal punishment is usually effective because pain is a universal language.

- So for **a baby 6 months old to 2 years old telling** them "no" and then giving them a tiny pinch on the arm/leg is usually effective. Now before you get angry with me remember that we give babies and kids VACCINES to protect them from illness, and a vaccine hurts MUCH more than a pinch right? So please no calls, texts or emails to Dr. Megan about being mean to babies.☹ The purpose is to instruct and correct a behavior that could harm them.

- **From 3 years old to 5 years old** you can probably spank using your hand or a little wooden spoon or plastic spatula. **NOTE:** *When I speak of spanking I want to be clear about what I mean: if the child has bruises/marks, is bleeding, limping and does not completely recover after 1 minute--meaning they are no longer crying and off playing again--then that is very likely ABUSE and **I DO NOT CONDONE ABUSE!** Do not spank in anger, it should be only to help teach and protect! Some people are strongly against corporal punishment and if you are that is fine. Just find some sort of discipline that is age appropriate and or effective and use that consistently.*
  Of course I was a model child and received very few spankings—but I did get some until I was about 10 years old and I turned out just fine if I say so myself! ☺ My mom was the spanker in our house. It is funny because my dad was the lecturer. He *never* spanked us but we ALL would have preferred if he had because he use to make us analyze and think about our bad behavior and it would take at least 30 minutes to an hour! Even as a 9 year old I remember thinking once while listening to one of my dad's lectures "man, this is 30 minutes of my life that I will never get back!"☹
  I willingly go to my parents for "lectures" now. Funny how the older you get, the less dumb you think your parents are! My parents are the ***best*** in the world though and I am very fortunate and grateful for them! ☺

- **From 6 years old to 10 years old** reasoning is greatly improved so you may not even need to spank at that point because they can understand that if they run into the street they might get hit by a car or that if they drink from the bottles under the sink it will make them sick. Discipline at that level could be "time out corners" or many other non-corporal methods.

- **11 years to 17 years** could be restriction of time with friends, electronics taken away etc. Be sure to make the punishment fit the "crime" and not have the same punishment for everything. **An undisciplined or "bratty" child will become a "bratty" undisciplined adult!** They do not grow out of it and they become a strain on society so please do not be lazy in this area. In addition, depending on your state or country where you live YOU can be called into question or even jailed for the actions of your child! Of course, if YOU the parent were never disciplined you will likely not know how to properly help your child and as I always say *"you cannot make a nice sandwich with two moldy pieces of bread"*. Therefore, **look for resources such as books on parenting or use counselors** to help you.

There are two television shows that have practical parenting tips. **One is "Supernanny with Jo Frost"** which is the **British version** and **"America's Supernanny"** with Deborah Tillman. Both women are trained experts! **These reality shows have EXCELLENT tips for disciplining and training children as well as helping parents correct the bad behaviors IN THEMSELVES that make their kids act crazy.** You can find these two on YouTube. Sometimes the networks show reruns: ABC for Supernanny and Lifetime network for America's Supernanny.

- **18 years and older** is when you enter more into the "friend" mode because you have already established the foundation for your child. Of course, if your adult child still lives under your roof then some of your rules may still apply. You are the King or Queen of your castle after all.☺

#2 You did or are doing your best to raise your kids so stop feeling guilty!
I have had parents literally crying about how and where they went wrong with raising their kids and these parents actually MAKE themselves sick blaming themselves about what they could have done better! Remember, as long as you loved your child and you tried your very best then YOU ARE or WERE a good parent! Now it is up to the child--especially at 18 years old and older--to make their own decisions whether GOOD or BAD and learn from them!
Stop blaming and judging yourself!

I was talking to a mom the other day and told her that if she could answer "yes" to any of the following questions then indeed she was a bad parent:

(1) Have you ever put your child's hands in boiling water?
(2) Did you ever try to sell your child on the internet?
(3) Have you ever told your child how dumb/ugly/unwanted they were?
(4) Did you purposefully deny your child food, clothing, shelter or education?
(5) Did you *KNOWINGLY* allow someone to physically, sexually or mentally/emotionally hurt your child?

She could not answer yes to any of those questions. So I told her that she was a good parent! These are TRUE examples of what some poor children have experienced! They tell me about it at their visits. ☹☹

If you as the parent/caregiver cannot answer yes to any of those questions above then pat yourself on the back and MOVE ON! ☺ If you did answer yes to one of these questions, at some point in your parenthood, then see chapter 8, Nature's Law number 7, and section 1 on "forgiveness".

ADVICE FOR COUPLES

Keep each other first!—Do not let any tangible thing, person or ideal separate you. Be sure to take care of each other and your couple FIRST before you run around putting work, your kids/parents or even doing GOOD things for other people before your couple time. Kids are important, but I often see parents separate or divorce once kids are older because as soon as they had kids the couple life became second to being parents. Mothers are notorious in forgetting that you were a woman and wife before you were mom! You are FIRST and FOREMOST a team of two, and teammates are always working together. Like on a basketball team, sometimes one member will be able to take a shot/make a goal more than another will, but then later they may have to switch for a time. Do not become proud if you are currently the team member making the most shots—for example earning the most money--because that could change in the future. On the other hand, do not be too proud to ALLOW the other person to take the shot/pass the ball, when you know that the other person is in a better position to take the shot! You always work for the greater short-term and long-term good of the team and keep individual stardom out of it!
THERE SHOULD BE NO COMPETITION IN LOVE AND COMMITMENT!

Communication!—Among two people of the same language and culture there can be misunderstanding particularly if they are from different backgrounds. The intention of what you are trying to say can EASILY be misunderstood if the two people are from different countries with different languages and cultures. What you mean to say can become "cloudy" when speaking. Therefore, no matter what background or country you are from, before becoming upset in a discussion/argument, do not pay attention to the <u>words</u> spoken but try to find the *intent* of what was said.

(1) Let the other person speak first. We all want to get our point across first. So each one is trying to talk at the same time and the conversation does not go well for either side. However, if you let the other person speak first--and truly listen to them and repeat to them what you understand that they are trying to say to you-- then they will feel heard and understood and will usually listen to you 100% when it is your turn to speak. I have seen this work OVER and OVER again!

(2) Ask for clarification, do not assume or interpret things—ask, "when you said this—did you mean (blank) or explain what you are trying to say again please". If you DO want to assume something then always try to assume that the person did or said something **<u>NOT</u> with the intent to hurt you or make you angry,** but to help/benefit you, since after all you are a team! *Of course if you know that you are in a relationship with a bad person then chances are they DID do or say something on purpose to hurt you.* ☹

(3) With disagreements/arguments limit and resolve them in the same DAY--do not stay mad for days on end; it becomes harder to remember exactly what was said (or done) and you keep your stress hormone Cortisol high for a long period. This will mess up Brain, Digestion and Heart cities! If you cannot continue to talk about the subject at the time, agree to take a break and establish a better time to finish discussing it. **One person is not always all right or the other person always all wrong so be prepared to assume at least 50% of any problem** that may arise, although sometimes it is more one person's fault than another's.

Example 1: A mother was angry with her adult child because she claims that the <u>adult child never calls</u> her. The adult child says that they do call their mother but they cannot call as often as the mother would like. The adult child added that the mother only calls the adult child when the <u>mother needs some chore</u> or service done around the house. Each one feels that the other is 100% wrong. Analyzing this situation, we could actually go back and look at phone records to see how many times each person called the other and indeed the adult child rarely called the mother over a period of months. Therefore, the adult child had to assume 50% being wrong that they should call more often. As for the mother, she had to assume 50% and recognize that she DID only call the adult child when she needed to ask for something to be done around the house. The mother came to understand that the adult child needs the mother to call the adult child just to check up on them and make sure the adult child is ok and not only call when she needs something. Do you see how this works?

Example 2: A wife is angry with her husband because he did not bring back the right box of bran cereal from the grocery store. The wife blames the husband telling him that he should have asked her the exact brand she wanted. The husband is mad at the wife because he brought back bran cereal as she asked and the wife never mentioned which brand she wanted and now instead of thanking him she is angry. Each one blames the other for 100% of the problem. Analyzing this example the wife should take 50% of the problem and recognize that she did not tell the husband which brand to get and that in the future she should give him a list or tell him which brand she wants.

The husband should take 50% of the problem and recognize that he could have asked if she wanted a specific brand before he left the house or at least tried to call her at the grocery store to check.

I know you think that this might be outside of what a visit to the doctor should be but when people sit down in front of me they begin talking about whatever last problem they had and I have to diffuse the situation so that I can get to the health part of their visit! In addition, we can see in a clinic settings how people's blood pressure can go VERY HIGH during the time of an argument or just after; so again these situations can then lead to a medical problem!

 It is in our nature to blame the other person for EVERYTHING and to want to be 100% in the right. However, we must PRACTICE ACTIVELY looking for areas where we are wrong or did not act in the best way and assume some percent of the problem.

- Avoid <u>definitive</u> criticism "you *never* OR *always* do/say (blank)"
- Avoid putting a person down, bad language, name calling
- Avoid becoming defensive when complaints are brought
- Avoid stonewalling/not speaking or using the "silent treatment"
- Avoid raising your voice or getting into each other's faces when upset
- Avoid throwing things, slamming doors, pointing fingers in faces
- Avoid leaving in the middle of an argument while someone is still talking

(4) Say you are sorry and be specific—if you do or say something wrong—whether it was on purpose or by mistake--apologize! Do not look for reasons why you were right. When apologizing be specific and do not simply say, "I am sorry".
Example: "I am sorry that when I called you lazy that I hurt your feelings". I was angry and I did not mean it. Of course, if you DO think that they are lazy, then do not lie and say that you do not. However, you can still say, "I am sorry because I know that when I called you lazy that probably made you feel badly". See how this works? Being specific helps the other person know that you understand exactly how your behavior hurt them. It is important to be VERY mindful of what you say to people when you are angry. Words last FOREVER; even though people may forgive you, they will still remember what you said. *What you said may be true,*

but how you said the words might have been mean. Once mean words leave your mouth you cannot bring them back in (like a sneeze) so take a deep breath before you speak angry words because you can really hurt someone you love by speaking too quickly! **A GREAT TRICK:** Just take a deep breath and call them whatever bad names or say what you want about them—but **do it IN YOUR HEAD NOT OUT LOUD**—that way you can still "say" what you want, but you do not hurt them and you avoid having to apologize later! ☺

(5) Make important decisions about finances, kids and life projects etc. when you are both at your best time to communicate. If one of you is a rooster and thinks best in the daytime, and one of you is an owl and thinks best late at night, do not try to have an important conversation at the other person's worst time. Try to find a time in the middle.

(6) In decision making try to do what is best individually for each member and for the team. This requires compromise. No one member will always be able to get 100% of what they want at the time so try to see how both of you can get MOST of what you want individually so that each person can walk away a little happy. Try to arrange things so that each of you gets approximately 50% of what you want. Sometimes, one of you may have only 49% while the other has 51%. My math is not strong but I believe this should add up to 100% right? ☺ Also, have all disagreements in any other room except the bedroom, this should be a place of harmony used only for sleep and sex (chick-a-pow pow!). ☺ So if you think your conversation is becoming an argument, make your way to the living room!

*Note: Being angry for whatever reason is very harmful to the body! A study done by The Institute of HeartMath[47] on medical students showed that **after just five minutes of anger** the participants IgA (Digestion city protection antibodies) decreased below the baseline for MORE THAN 6 HOURS! That means you are not handling food well or getting the vitamins or minerals as you should. Nor is your immune system/police in the United States of You working well for 6 HOURS!* **Can you imagine the amount of crime that would happen in your city of residence if the criminals knew that the police were "on break" for 6 hours?!?** *Obviously we cannot avoid being angry all of the time, but let us make sure that we are doing our best not to be angry over truly stupid things--traffic, spouse forgot to take out the trash--and reserve our anger for more important things like racism, social injustices, abuse of the small and weak.*

However, please do try to remember to take out the trash regularly because having too much trash in the house is nasty.☹

Discuss and set clear boundaries about what is acceptable behavior with regard to cheating. Discuss what exactly "cheating" would constitute—flirting, just talking on the phone, hand holding, kissing etc. You may think a kiss on the mouth is cheating and your spouse really may not think so because they may think that only having sex would be cheating. Discuss physical cheating versus emotional cheating. **Example physical cheating:** one heterosexual couple (man and woman) went for counseling because of infidelity/cheating. The man was angry that the woman had cheated on him by kissing someone else. The woman did not think that she had really cheated because the person she kissed was another woman. The woman in the couple did not identify herself as a lesbian, she was not attracted to the other woman she kissed. She was just curious to see what it was like to kiss another woman. The man felt she cheated because she kissed someone else and he did not care whether it was a man or woman. You see how this can create a huge problem? This is why you must discuss these topics very specifically.

 Example emotional cheating: I have seen couples where one person may not think that sharing very personal details of their lives--including details on their romantic relationship with another person (over a long period of time) is cheating. Your spouse or partner may think that it is emotional cheating; especially if the person that you are sharing information with is of the opposite sex or might like you romantically. Even in committed but "open" relationships where people are exclusively dating or married but allow each other to see other people, eventually one person will get angry about how often the other person is seeing other people and so it usually will break the couple apart. My advice is if you are single, be single. If you are married or committed, then be in the couple and keep extra people out of it. If you have couple problems and you really need to discuss it with someone then usually a family member is the better option. I have seen best friends cheat with each other's wives/husbands/partners etc. The cheating usually occurs with someone in your circle not with a perfect stranger. Less drama is always best. ☺ This way you can avoid having to go to the emergency room because your spouse or partner stabbed you with a fork at dinner.☹

(7) Say thank you! These two little words make ANY person feel appreciated! Yes, perhaps it is your partner's responsibility to cut the grass and cook. However, it is still nice to be thanked for doing something EVEN if you are supposed to do it! Saying thank you is VERY important in a couple but you can use these words for everyone really. Thank your kids for doing their homework or chores. Thank your boss for paying you.☺

(8) Stay in shape for your spouse or partner—**Women:** we cannot use the excuse of carrying children as a reason to allow ourselves to stay out of shape. Try to get back to your pre-baby size or fairly close. It is possible! Celebrities do it all the time! Yes, they do have personal chefs and personal trainers but they still must do the work themselves to lose the weight. Your spouse/partner will usually accept you heavier though so do not use unhealthy methods to accomplish this goal. Do not go crazy trying to get to a certain size either. Balance is important!

Men: realize that indeed, it is not easy to carry a baby and that it will wreak havoc onto a woman's body. Boobs/breasts and bum/rear end tend to travel "south" and the stomach and hips travel "east and west" meaning they get wider; not to mention the mental and emotional changes. Try to be supportive throughout and after this process. Additionally, do not overdo on food/beer/soda and "grow" a large stomach so that *you* look 9 months pregnant yourself.☹

Men and Women: if you have gained weight for another reason then it is time to get back into tune with Nat 9 so that you can maintain a healthy size. You can see chapter 11 "Doc, help me lose weight" for help.

(9) Maintain a healthy sexual life. Many things may affect your intimate life but it is usually a physical, mental/emotional or underlying disease/medical condition.

- **Physical problems** such as a back, neck or other injury or limitation.
- **Mental/emotional problems** such as if you have a negative view about sexual relations—this could stem from sexual abuse in childhood/adult or develop for some other reason. You may have a negative view of your body after pregnancy or surgery.
- **Underlying disease or medical problems** such as Diabetes or high blood pressure in a man can make it difficult for him to achieve or maintain an erection or in woman after menopause the decrease in Estrogen and Progesterone can make vaginal intercourse painful.

After childbirth, hormone levels can change and make a woman lose desire for sex. Medications can decrease libido/sex drive in both men and women.

The idea here is to not just leave your spouse "high and dry" or without intimacy because of your health problem. You are a team, therefore you owe it to them, and to yourself to maintain your sexual life as much as is possible while you are searching to improve your health. For example, if you have a back injury and cannot engage in full intercourse in a certain position then try another, or play "hand games" or improvise! Use "toys"! I am trying to keep this section vague since I did intend for this to be a family or rated "PG" book.☺ However, I hope you understand what I mean here? Do not just say to yourself or to your spouse or partner I am sick/injured and so I cannot do ANYTHING and just avoid or eliminate sexual activity. Actively search to get your health back on track and in the meantime keep "playing" with your spouse and partner in creative ways based on your current ability! You do not want to become "roommates" or "platonic" friends! You are in a romantic relationship--no matter how old you both get--so act like it! Chik-a-pow pow! ☺ If it is a relationship of convenience--for legal or financial gain--and not based on love/romance then just ignore all that I said.

Note: in the case of women who have intimacy problems because of vaginal changes that come with menopause, you can ask your doctor about taking a compounded hormonal cream with the Estrogens, Progesterone and Testosterone and apply that topically to the area so that it can help it to retake form a little bit. Taking oral bioidentical hormones as a replacement can be an option as well. However, make sure that your health care professional is prescribing hormones in levels that would approximately match what you should normally have around your age. It can be very dangerous for your health if you are using **(1)** non-bio identical hormones because they are foreign to the body and will cause bad side effects or **(2)** using bioidentical hormones at levels that are abnormal for your stage in life.

 Example: if you are a 50-year-old woman then you want to take all the appropriate hormones at levels that your body would have made just before menopause at 40 or 45 years old. Meaning you should not use a prescription for oral or topical hormones that take your hormone levels back to what they were when you were 25 years old! That is going too far against nature. Does this make sense? Make sure you double and triple check this with your health professional because sadly this mistake is often made with hormonal prescriptions.

For women it is usually with Estrogen and Progesterone prescriptions and for men it is with Testosterone prescriptions. **Going too far away from nature gives us SERIOUS side effects and health problems!** ☹

If there is no injury or medical problem with the act of being intimate then periodically remember to try new and fun "games" together! Be open about communicating games you would like to try and games that you no longer like or if you are a little bored with certain things. Your spouse/partner is probably not a mind reader so be open about what you like or do not like. Be sure to make a request in a nice way. Here is an example "can we try this (insert game here) instead?" and NOT "I hate it when you do this"! Usually it is best not to make mention of things you do not like while you are in the middle of that particular game so that your spouse/partner does not feel ashamed or embarrassed. Tell them before or sometime after. Although if you feel you must make a tiny correction in the middle of a game then again, do it very sweetly. As long as you are both comfortable with the activity then is should be ok.

Things to Avoid: (1) putting random objects in to any "holes" of the body. Particularly objects with moving parts or small pieces that can break and or get "lost". This likely will end in a hospital visit. **(2)** using chemicals such as gels, dyes, lotions, and certain food products in sensitive areas (again around any holes) because this will DEFINITELY result in a hospital visit. ☹ **(3)** be very careful if being intimate outside in nature. Insects and creepy, crawly things are always looking for nice, warm, moist holes to crawl into. No further explanation needed.☹☹

There are many resources out there on the Internet, in libraries and counselors to help you both in this area. Sexuality is another area where you should be "studying" to become the best student you can for your spouse/partner!

(10) Do not wait for the other person to "fail". An example of "waiting for someone to fail is thinking to yourself "let me see if my spouse/partner remembers my birthday/Valentine's day/our anniversary this year, because they forgot last year". Therefore, if they do indeed forget again you are very prepared to yell at them. Instead, help them succeed! A week or two before the event tell them "Guess what? My birthday/Valentine's Day/our anniversary is coming up soon and I would really love for you to plan a surprise or a party for me or to give me this certain gift".

That way instead of spending the day of the event mad at your partner or spouse because they forgot AGAIN just as you knew they would, you can spend it happy and enjoying the day together.☺

Couples Counseling

Do not wait until things go wrong. Once every 3 months or so, go together to see a marriage/couples counselor where you can talk things over and just make sure that you both are feeling good about where you are as a couple. Often it is easier to express certain feelings in front of a third person than between the two of you. The counselor can give you ideas on how to make your couple stronger and happier!

Remember to have fun! Make each other feel loved and wanted, respect each other's individual identity and maintain your own separate friends. Do fun things together, have new experiences! Support each other's goals and dreams and work towards them together! It does not cost anything to dream! Just make sure you are still putting food on the table though.☺

I said that this advice was for couples but really, we could apply these principles to ANY relationship: parent to child, between brothers or sisters and even between friends or coworkers...well all principles can apply except the one about sexual activity of course...that one still ONLY applies for romantic relationships.☺

RESOURCE: Books and DVDs by Mark Gungor[65] called **"Laugh Your Way to a Better Marriage".** These are very funny and are practical for couples. You can also find the videos on YouTube to get a preview.

RESOURCE: Book: **"The Five Love Languages"** by Gary Chapman.[66]Explains how we express and receive love. Very insightful for ANY type relationship! Not only romantic. He also has the same type book as it relates to kids and teens.

These books are perfectly in tune with the experiences I have lived as well as in an office setting working with couples. These books are by Christian authors, however if you are not a Christian do not worry, they are not very Christian-y. The principles pertain to human behavior and apply to everyone! No matter what religion or creed or the absence thereof.☺

ADVICE FOR SINGLE PEOPLE Teens and 20's. Drugs, Alcohol and Dating.

This is usually the time when people make the STUPIDEST decisions of their lives that will affect them medically either in the present or in the future so I wanted to add a little blurb here for you guys. **I have a saying "Don't do "stupid" stupidly!** That means that if you are doing an activity that is harmful to you or someone else (therefore it is stupid) DO NOT engage in that activity in the worse possible way so that you will increase the already bad effect on you or others (stupidly):

Drugs and Alcohol
I do not advocate the use of either street drugs or alcohol alone; and it is ESPECIALLY dangerous to use them together because if you do use one or both then you will put yourself (and others) at an increased risk of entering into the medical system in some way!

Patient 1: Young girl in her 20's who went on a trip out of the country and got really drunk and slept with a stranger, now in the office crying in front of me because she is scared she is pregnant and does not want a baby right now--especially since she has no clue who the dad is--and she is in college and working.

Common examples that often happen with too much alcohol:
- Unplanned pregnancies--nearly half of the pregnancies in the U.S. are unplanned
- Driving under the influence (DUI) resulting in death or injury to yourself or others
- MEN: being beaten, stabbed, shot and or killed
- WOMEN: being raped, beaten, stabbed, shot and or killed
- BOTH: being arrested...that is legal, not medical...but still worth mentioning.

Don't do stupid stupidly: if you are going to drink, do not drink to the point of being drunk! Why not? You no longer have full function of your mind and will make VERY bad choices that will affect you and others for years to come! Not to mention the damage done to your poor liver and kidneys.
- **If you do want to drink to the point of being completely drunk "wasted/trashed" then DO THAT AT HOME with your friends!** At least everyone stays safe! Or if you must go out, assign a non-drinking friend (or pay someone) to be your "body guard" who watches you and makes sure you do not do anything stupid like go home with a stranger or get into some bad situation where you might be hurt or taken advantage of.
- **Women especially must guard against high use of alcohol** because we have less enzymes that break down alcohol than men do. So women, in general, will get drunk faster than men will. Some nationalities such as Asian women, have the least alcohol enzymes amongst all women so they can really get drunk quickly. *Analogy: remember the beginning of the book with the monkey? The monkey (enzyme) is in a room and we throw handfuls of bananas (alcohol) into*

the room for him to try to peel them and eat them as fast as he can. As long as he can keep up with peeling and eating bananas at a fast rate then all is well and you will not get drunk. But if unpeeled bananas are building up in the room then you are getting drunk. Men have more alcohol enzymes than women so that is as if men have TWO or THREE monkeys in their room peeling bananas while women only have one monkey. Does it make sense?

- **Women again:** do not accept drinks (even nonalcoholic) from strangers. Do not leave your drink unattended OR turn your back to your drink. Do not allow bartenders to prepare your drink with their back turned to you, meaning you cannot see what their hands are doing. These are just classic ways that women are drugged and raped whether it is in a bar or at a house party. Do not allow friends to get drinks for you either because perhaps the friend was not paying attention to what the bartender was doing. Be super alert in these areas!

BIRTH CONTROL OPTIONS/CONTRACEPTION

The first patient was a girl who feared an unplanned pregnancy so this seemed to be a good place to talk about the different ways to prevent pregnancy. Typically, a gynecologist and potentially a urologist (men) would have more detailed information on the different forms possible and their benefits and side effects. Please consult a gynecologist for the latest information on contraception.

When contemplating the different forms of contraception, it is important to be well informed. Factors to consider when contemplating contraception:

(1) Financial resources

(2) Pattern/frequency of sexual intercourse

(3) Risk of sexually transmitted illness/STI

(4) Desire to maintain future fertility/baby making possibilities

(5) Access to medical care

The forms of contraception/birth control are:
(1) Hormonal: oral and non-oral
(2) Barrier methods
(3) Fertility awareness/Fertility planning
(4) Tubal Ligation; Essure* or Vasectomy* (men)
 * *these involve surgery and are permanent contraception.*

Note: WOMEN your menstrual cycle* and or menses/periods* are abnormal if:

- your cycle comes less than every 21 days or more than every 35 days
- your period lasts less than 3 days or more than 8 days
- you have heavy bleeding meaning you are changing pads/tampons hourly or else you are bleeding through clothes or bedding
- you barely bleed at all; meaning you could wear one pad/tampon all day long without having to change it--*obviously we want to change more often for hygiene but I am speaking of how much blood flows*
- you have spotting/drops of blood between periods
- you have strong pain that makes you double over or have to lie in bed
- you have nausea, vomiting, or headaches/migraines
- you have to take a day(s) off work or school every cycle
- you have to take medications for pain or other symptoms

I mean a natural cycle/period. If you are on birth control it will change your cycle.

If you have any of the issues above you need to work on balancing your hormones and cleaning out Liver city--from a Chinese medicine perspective.

- It is *common* for **women to have horrible periods** but it is **not normal**.
- Your period should be between painless and mildly uncomfortable.
- **Your period should not be the Apocalypse.**☹

Taking medications that reduce your cycle to a few times a year or stop your cycle completely is bad! Whether you take a cycle changing medication for convenience—I know, no one wants a period--or to avoid pain and suffering, it goes AGAINST NATURE and you are ASKING for HEALTH TROUBLES!

Analogy 1: *that is like the smallest, weakest kid in the school going up to the biggest, strongest kid in the school and calling him stupid! Asking for trouble!*

Analogy 2: *imagine the electricity was functioning abnormally in your house. The lights turn on and off at random times. You would not just tell the electric company to disconnect the electricity completely would you? NO! Because it is an important part of the house.*

You would instead have the electrician look for the problem and fix it!

Likewise with your cycle. It is part of women's health! You cannot just "turn it off".

HORMONAL-ORAL

This is the use of Estrogens and/or Progestins to "trick" the body into thinking it is already pregnant. Choice of a pill--your gynecologist should obtain your full medical history and physical exam: blood pressure, breast exam, pelvic exam, pap smear, liver functions, family and social history. They should ask your age at first menstrual cycle, regularity and length of cycle and periods, date of last period, spotting, premenstrual syndrome/PMS, birth control use history, including side effects and compliance.

Daily Use
- Estrogen and Progestin Combination pill (COC)
- Extended cycle pill
- Progestin only pill (POP)

Non-daily use
- Injectable
- Contraceptive patch
- Vaginal ring
- Hormone--releasing intrauterine (inside the uterus) system

Since the prescription hormone activity is either greater or less than the hormone effect of a woman's own natural ovarian hormones, typical **side effects:**

- Bleeding irregularities--32%
- Nausea--19%
- Weight gain--14%
- Mood swings--14%
- Breast tenderness--11%
- Headache--11%
- Decrease in libido/sex drive

Less common but more serious side effects/risks of inappropriate or prolonged use of hormonal oral contraceptives are **(1)** blood clots which can lead to: stroke, heart attack, blockage of blood vessels in the lungs and **(2)** potential development of cancer--notably in the breast* *again speak with gynecologist about risk factors.*

They can also interact with other medications notably: anticonvulsant/seizure medications, antibiotics, antifungals, sedatives/sleep medications and botanical medications. **WARNING:** certain antibiotics can interfere with your oral birth control and make it stop working! So if you get an infection while on birth control be sure to verify with the doctor prescribing the antibiotic to see if it will interact with your birth control.

HORMONAL NON-ORAL

Contraceptive patch (Ortho Evra)--99% effective

- Applied weekly (3 weeks on, 1 week off)
- **Disadvantages:** skin irritation, slightly higher incidence of breast tenderness and nausea reported; increased risk for blood clots. A study links the patch to more than doubling the risk for blood clots/traffic jams in the legs!

Contraceptive ring (Nuva Ring)

- Applied monthly (3 weeks on, 1 week off)
- **Disadvantages:** Vaginal discomfort reported, but rare. Potential expulsion/body pushes out device and insertion technique is hard

Progestin only Implants

- Does not affect lactation/breast feeding
- Ovulation/egg traveling returns in 50% of women within three months and almost 90% within in one year.
- Must take it every day at the same time of day. If more than 3 hours late taking the pill, must use a second method of contraception until the next period
- **Side Effects:**
  - Unpredictable spotting and breakthrough bleeding, occasional loss of period
  - With Depo-Provera--irregular bleeding, loss of period is common.
  - Headache, mood changes, weight gain, decreases in HDL "good cholesterol"and increases in LDL "bad cholesterol". **Note:** LDL is not truly bad. We need LDL cholesterol, just not too much.

Implanon

- An implanted form of Progestin--only birth control
- A matchstick-sized rod is implanted in a woman's upper arm, where it releases a slow but steady stream of synthetic/fake Progesterone for up to three years.
- Works similarly to Norplant, but a different form of Progesterone at a lower dose.
- Some may have the same side effects as they did with Norplant: abnormal uterine bleeding, loss of period
- **Side Effects:** weight gain, headache, mood swings, acne, and depression. Not recommended if there is a history of blood blots, unexplained vaginal bleeding, liver disease, or breast cancer.
- Effectiveness: less than one pregnancy per 100 women who use it for one year.

BARRIER METHODS

Effectiveness can vary on proper insertion, weight gain/loss, type of spermicide used or not used etc. Percentages listed below are approximate:

- **Diaphragm** with spermacide-81-98% effective; **FemCap** with spermicide is 88-98% effective; **Sponge**-79-91% effective
- **Condoms** (male-85-98% effective;female-79-95% effective)
- **Spermicides**: 79-97% effective in killing sperm-Nonoxynol-9 is an example

Please speak with a gynecologist/urologist for more detailed information, but general barrier method **risks and side effects:**

- Toxic Shock Syndrome-bacteria build up on the material and get in blood→systemic infection! ☹ LIFE THREATENING. Not very common.
- Sexually Transmitted Illnesses (STI)
- Pregnancy ☹
- Irritation and/or inflammation of the vaginal tissues or penis
- Urinary tract infections
- Allergy to device materials (like to the latex in condoms) or spermicides

FERTILITY AWARENESS

Fertility Awareness relies upon the following assumptions:

- Sperm can live in a woman's body up to 5 days after intercourse, though more often 2 days. ***Pregnancy is most likely to happen if intercourse occurs anywhere from 3 days before ovulation-when the egg moves from the ovaries/egg holding room to the uterus/baby hotel-until 2-3 days after ovulation*** ☹

Works by monitoring changes in your body that indicate you *will* ovulate/release an egg or are ovulating *right now*. Means your chance is higher to get pregnant.

- Basal Body Temperature-generally there is an increase in temperature at ovulation
- Cervical mucus--is thinner during ovulation
- Ovulation predictor kits/Lutenizing Hormone(LH) kit--LH is higher during ovulation
- Difficulty: irregular menses can make this a very difficult process
- **Side effects:** pregnancy ☹

SURGICAL PROCEDURES:

Tubal ligation; Essure; Vasectomy (men)

Tubal Ligation—having your "tubes tied"
- 98% effective
- Tubal ligation is permanent closing of the fallopian tubes. Fallopian tubes are cut, burned, or blocked with rings, bands or clips so they no longer have a connection to the uterus/baby hotel.
- Typically has no effect on sexual function or desire.*
- Generally should not change the monthly menstrual cycle or menopause.*
- Performed laparoscopically and usually done under general anesthesia.
- May resume intercourse usually within one week after surgery
- May be reversible 60-80%

side effects/after effects: happens rarely, but a woman could still become pregnant after the procedure!☹ Also not typical, but after surgery scarring in the area can affect menstrual cycle: heavy bleeding causing fainting and anemia/low red blood cells/semi-trucks, and reducing normal blood flow in that area as well as changes in libido/sex drive and mental or emotional changes. Each person may react differently since every person is a unique individual.

Essure
- Irreversible surgical procedure without the need for an abdominal incision or general anesthesia
- An Essure micro-insert is placed in each fallopian tube/baby making tunnel. The micro-insert expands upon release, anchoring itself in the fallopian tube. The micro-insert then makes a benign natural tissue response. Tissue in-growth into the micro-insert permanently holds the device in place and closes up the fallopian tube, resulting in sterilization/an egg road block.
- The Essure system was 99.80% effective after 4 years of follow up and has been demonstrated to be 99.74% effective at 5 years follow up.
- **What You Should Know:** Backup birth control must be used for three months, after which a test is done to check how open the fallopian tube is.
- Studies show blockage is substantial/pretty good at three months and increases at six months

Remember: a girl or woman only has a certain number of eggs. She already has these eggs in her ovaries/egg holding room while SHE is still a baby in her mom! Once a girl enters puberty, every month an egg will leave the ovaries/egg holding room and travel through the fallopian tubes/baby making tunnel. If a sperm from dad is traveling along the same "tunnel" at the same time as the egg, then the sperm and egg will join and become the future baby. The future baby then travels down to the uterus/baby hotel and grows for nine months. Then mom pushes out the baby. On the other hand, if the egg does not meet a sperm traveling through the fallopian tubes/baby making tunnel then the egg will keep on traveling and eventually fall out of the girl/woman's body. This is the menstrual cycle/period. The process will start over again the next month and occur in this way until the woman loses all of her eggs. That is menopause/ran out of eggs time. At this point, the woman can no longer have a baby. ***Analogy:*** *you cannot make an omelet without eggs!* Tee. Hee. I am so clever sometimes. Ok. I know that was cheesy. Hey! Omelets can have cheese too! I am on a joke roll. Someone stop me! ☺

VASECTOMY (men)
- 99% effective
- The vas deferens are cut and closed either by sewing them or putting surgical clips on the end of each of the vas deferens thereby preventing sperm from being able to travel.
- **PROS:** Procedure is 30 minutes under local anesthesia. Recovery from vasectomy usually requires only that the patient refrain from heavy physical activity for approximately 48 hours.
- **CONS:** Complications are relatively rare, but can involve bleeding and infection, swelling of the scrotum/holds the testes=the sperm holding room, and change in function in the area. Potential link to prostate cancer. Success rate for reversal is low.

Be thoroughly informed when making a decision about contraception because if not, the side effects could be a decrease in health and wellness and/or pregnancy.☹ **Having a child is a lifelong "side effect" if you did not plan for it. You are a parent until you die or the child dies. They did not ask to be born! Therefore, you should not enter into parenthood casually!** Be sure to exhaust all informational avenues and find a gynecologist/urologist/health care practitioner that will assist you in your goals.

Drugs and Alcohol continued
Story: this was not a patient of mine but still a sad story I heard. A girl goes out to a bar and has some drinks and she blacks out. She wakes up the next day naked, in a field surrounded by condoms. **WOMEN third time:** we are generally less able to defend ourselves against physical attacks EVEN with full use of our senses but we are especially at risk when we are drinking or using drugs! I am not justifying rape (or any kind of abuse) of a person. It is wrong to hurt anyone, young or old, male or female whether the person is conscious/unconscious/drugged out or drunk. What I want to beg young women to do here though, is to not make it EASY for someone to hurt you! Rape has very long lasting mental, emotional and physical effects on a person.☹

Note: I focus more on women here simply because men are typically only at <u>high</u> risk of rape when they are in prison. However, the negative effects of rape are the same whether the victim is a woman, man, adult or child.

Analogy: we know that burglars exist, so do not leave your front door open so that they can just WALK in! Lock your doors! Get an alarm system, maybe a dog too! Likewise, when drinking PLEASE, PLEASE be on top of your "game" and stay at level orange high alert! Most women are raped by someone that they know and not by a perfect stranger. Meaning by an acquaintance: someone they just met or by a "friend" so be very careful at someone else's house party, but also at bars or where ever.

- **If you are drinking, then EAT** also because this will slow down the absorption of alcohol into your system. Crackers, chips just whatever.
- **Do not drink or taste someone else's drink.** You never know what is in it (drugs for them or to drug you) or they may have some disease that you can catch just by drinking after them. This also applies to water bottles!
- **DO NOT DRINK AND DRIVE!** Hire someone (a friend is best) to be the non-drinking person and have them drive. It is very unfair for you to go out and have a nice time partying and then get in the car and paralyze, scar or kill <u>someone else</u> because of your drunk driving! If you want to hurt yourself in some way that is your choice. Drive to a cliff and drink all you want and then drive off the cliff. Truly, I am not advocating this, but I hope you understand my point. You will hurt ONLY YOURSELF! The REST OF US want to be SAFE on the road.
- **Be careful with your cell phones.** They carry all of your personal information and can easily be used to by hooligans to follow you home etc.
- **Your house parties.** Invite only people you know WELL, do not make it a block party or allow your friends to invite people you do not know. That way it is less likely that someone will be beaten, raped, stabbed or shot.
- **Go out with <u>responsible</u> friends.** There is safety in numbers so look out for each other. Hopefully at least ONE of your friends can help you from doing something stupid or from being hurt.

Too much alcohol can really mess up Liver city and lead to many medical problems in the present as well as in the future. Notably in men, it can lead to erectile difficulties, which can be very embarrassing and frustrating when your "weenie" will not work! In women, it can mess up your menstrual cycle, which can lead to fertility problems. If you were already pregnant and did not know it yet, then you can damage the baby and make it mentally retarded or make them have problems in many areas of their body! Again, do not ruin your life (or even worse someone else's life) because of your partying!

Patient 2: young man in his late teens went to a party and took many drugs and slept with 6 people (that he remembers...could have been more) and did not use condoms. Now he is sitting in front of me very scared that he has a sexually transmitted disease/illness (STD/STI). **Note:** STD/STI is the same thing.

Don't do stupid stupidly: In this case, if this young man would have been in his right mind and he really wanted to sleep with 6 or more people then he would have thought to use condoms! Sexually transmitted illnesses/STIs do not only affect your Reproduction city they can affect ANY area of the body in the present or in the future! *Analogy: if a burglar breaks into your house using the living room window, does he just steal what is in the living room such as the flat screen TV, stereo or sound system? NO! He will go through the ENTIRE house and steal everything from everywhere!* This is how bacteria or viruses from STDs work also! They may enter the United States of You via reproduction areas but they will go to Liver, Brain and Musculoskeletal cities so that you may even have difficulty walking!

- **Drugs.** If you are going to use drugs, it is best not to use drugs that have a *high* capacity to change how well your mind works! Drugs such as cocaine, heroin etc. or even chemical products lying around the house that you can sniff/inhale will make you less able to make good decisions. Marijuana usually has the least affects. Again, I am not advocating or saying "yes" to drug use so please no calls or emails from mad parents please.☹

- **Protect yourself and <u>ALWAYS</u> wear condoms!** They will not protect you at 100% because they can break/tear but they are better than nothing! The Centers for Disease Control and Prevention (CDC) reports that nearly half of Americans have had sex with *at least two people* by the time they are 17 years old and that people are only using condoms <u>half</u> of the time! You do the math on how many people you really slept with when you sleep with ONE person without a condom. The number is exponential! Then think about all of the possible diseases! ☹

- **STD testing before you sleep with someone and periodically afterwards!** Remember that young man who slept with many people without using a condom? He is not the exception! <u>Therefore, I recommend this for singles as well as married or committed couples</u>. People can be carriers of STDs and *not have any symptoms* but they can infect YOU and <u>you</u> get symptoms! Therefore, you cannot always tell by just looking. You might think asking for an STD test will kill the romance, but so will having an STD!

161

It may help keep people honest too if they know every six months or so we are both doing a little "check". Infidelity/cheating is very common and can still happen even amongst couples who love each other!

HOT: A healthy weenie/penis OR va-gee-gee/vagina.☺
NOT HOT: pus oozing warts all over your weenie OR little bugs crawling around on your va-gee-gee.☹

Story: this was not a patient of mine but another sad story I heard. A young woman went to a bar and got a headache while she was there. She was not drinking though. A stranger offered her an Aspirin. She took the Aspirin from him, but did not want to take the pill at the bar so she returned home and then took the Aspirin there. She went to sleep and woke up the next day not knowing who she was. Her long-term memory was almost completely erased! It was not an Aspirin that he gave her even though she had seen him pull it out of an Aspirin bottle.

Don't do stupid stupidly. As for the young woman, she <u>was not</u> using drugs or alcohol she really just made a very poor decision that involved a drug.☹

- **Drugs.** DO NOT TAKE <u>ANY PILLS OF ANY KIND</u> from ANYONE. ESPECIALLY NOT FROM STRANGERS or ACQUAINTANCES.
- **Medications.** This is a nice place for me to repeat that it is dangerous for you to take your mom's/dad's or friends prescribed medications! Even if they have acne and you have acne that does not mean you should take their medications for your acne! Medications are prescribed for THAT person and we take into account the overall health of the person.
  Analogy*: taking someone else's medication is like trying to change a flat tire on a bicycle by using a car tire! Yes they are both tires but one tire is specific to the bike and the other tire is specific to the car.* There are even <u>differences between two car tires</u>! You must match the tire to the vehicle!

Dating
The person that you have a romantic relationship with can have a HUMONGOUS impact on your health therefore it is very important to be wise about who you choose to date short-term and or long-term. A few pointers:
- **Desperate and lonely attract overbearing and mediocre:** If you are sending out "energy" into the "universe" that you are desperate and lonely for a romantic partner you will usually attract an overbearing person. Someone abusive; or you will attract a mediocre person: meaning someone lazy or unwilling to work or better himself or herself as a person. You may

even attract someone who will neglect you. There is truth in the old saying **"It is better to be alone than in bad company"**. Instead of focusing on what you do not have, fill your life with friends, work, purpose and other good things and just watch and see how the "universe" brings your future partner when the timing is right for you to receive them! If you are constantly going from relationship to relationship you may want to get counseling to see where the problem lies inside of you. You may be trying to fill an empty space that someone else left open such as your dad not being around, your mom not understanding you or your children hating you.

- **Masculine mindset versus the Feminine mindset.** Men and woman truly think differently. Most women (60% or more) will have the feminine mindset and most men will have the masculine mindset. However, you can have women with the masculine mindset and men with the feminine mindset. I will use the words "women" or "men" however, I am speaking about the mindset. It is very important to understand these differences in thinking so that there are no misunderstandings that then result in bad feelings. **(1)** Men are typically more stimulated by sight than women are. That is why men must usually find a woman attractive to date them. Whereas women can originally not find a man handsome, but then become attracted to him later because of how he makes her feel.

  Example: *look at all of the supermodels dating ugly men.* So essentially most men begin with physical/sexual attraction (south or private parts) and then fall in love (north or the heart/emotions) while most women begin with the heart (north) and then follows physical/sexual attraction (south). Most men do not need to be in love or even know the person in order to have sexual relations. They can separate the south from the north. Indeed, as long as a man finds the person attractive they can even HATE them but put that hatred aside long enough to be intimate. Women typically cannot be intimate with a person that they do not already love or at least care about deeply, even if they find them attractive. They definitely cannot sleep with someone that they dislike or hate unless they are forced. Women in general do not separate the north from the south.

Example: *the prostitution/trafficking industry is predominantly males exploiting women. You do not find women out looking to sleep with numerous random or unknown men.* **(2)** Most men want to feel strong, intelligent and desired sexually. Therefore, a person that is masterful at making him feel this way can convince him to do good OR bad things.

Example: <u>many</u> *crafty women have convinced men to commit crimes including murder for them!* On the other hand, most women want to feel beautiful, loved and protected. For that, reason women will often stay with a man who is at best mediocre or at worst physically or mentally abusive because the woman would rather have a man in their lives/feel protected than to be alone/unprotected. Women will often down play intelligence or accomplishments if they think the man feels threatened or does not like a girl to be too smart.

Advice for women/feminine mindset: Understand that a man can sleep with you even though he no longer loves you, or if he never loved or liked you to begin with. Do not confuse sex and love! This includes divorcing/committed couples that are breaking up! If a man tells you he no longer loves you, believe him! Do not think that because he can still sleep with you he must still love you. Therefore, unless you have agreed to be "friends with benefits", realize that the relationship is over. Unlike women, men tend to be very "black or white" when it comes to emotions. Either they love you or they do not. Women have more "grey" with our emotions and change a little from time to time. Many women ignore what men say about not loving them anymore if they are still sleeping together.

Be very clear about boundaries and what void you are trying to fill. Do not just look for someone to care for you but understand that you can care for yourself! You are beautiful, no matter what you look like! Do not downplay your personality, achievements or any other aspect of yourself for a romantic partner. The person should love and respect you for who you are!

Advice for men/masculine mindset: Be very clear about your intentions with dating. Are you dating with the intentions of forming a long-term relationship or is this only short-term? Most women are looking for a long-term commitment. Do not mislead or give false hope by calling/texting/hanging out/sleeping with a woman you are not truly interested in. After the first date, typically you already have an idea of how you feel about them with regard to a long-term relationship. If you are not looking for a long-term relationship then be honest and let them know. Realize that most women will become <u>VERY</u> clingy once you sleep with them. Therefore, it is best not to sleep with them if you are not serious.

Example: when a woman discovers that a man TRULY does not love her anymore or that he never liked her but has just been sleeping with her for the fun of it, she may turn violent in some way. This will likely end in a hospital visit or at least destruction of the man's personal property—usually his car☹. Perhaps you have heard the saying **"Hell hath no fury like a woman scorned"**. In other words, after someone pushes a woman too far in a negative direction, you had better watch out because you are in trouble! There have been multiple news stories where a woman ran over her cheating ex-man with her car...twice. Hospital visit. ☹

Note: men in general are more prone to violence than women are. Men initiate physical fights amongst themselves more often than women fight physically with other women. However, <u>when a woman turns violent</u> she will usually be MUCH meaner, <u>more calculating and creative with the violent act</u> than a man would be.☹

True story: when I was about 8 years old my brother A pulled off my Barbie doll's head and threw the head onto the roof of the house. I did not have many toys and my Barbies were <u>my favorite and most sacred</u> of toys. *I was enraged!* Fortunately for him, the head rolled back down the roof onto the ground because I could have literally killed him in that moment; even though he was eight years *older* than me and *much bigger*. But since the head fell back down, I decided to just teach him a lesson instead. I knew that he usually did not wear shoes around the house. So, I put two rows of nails along the bottom step, at the end of the staircase. Then I hid behind the wall next to the staircase and called his name. He came running down barefoot--as I knew he would--and when he reached that bottom step he started hopping up and down from one foot to the other saying "ooo" "aaa" "yoww" like a monkey. At the time I laughed and then threatened him that more "evil plans" would follow if he EVER messed with my Barbies again! ☹ Fortunately, the nails were dull so he did not get seriously hurt. **I am very sorry NOW that I did this because I loved him then and love him now too of course! Please kids (or adults) do not repeat this at home!** This just gives you a notion of how devious I was at 8 years old! Imagine the crazy things I could concoct now! ☹ I have not done any crazy thing since then ☺ but I could...☹ Just kidding! ☺ Sort of...☹. I repeat **MEN**: we woman can act crazy! Do not push us too far! When you play with a woman's emotions *you will be sorry*!
Oh, and my brother did not touch Barbie again. ☺

Advice for men/masculine mindset continued...
Do not commit heinous crimes or spend an inordinate amount of money or time on a conniving or materialistic woman! Women can be masterful at using their "charms" to get you to act very stupidly! No woman is worth legal or ethical troubles. There are plenty of nice, grounded people to date or marry. Beware of women who only want you for what you can give them!

For both mindsets: to truly know and understand someone else you must FIRST understand and know YOURSELF. How you think, your values, what makes you react in certain ways and in certain situations. How are your childhood experiences affecting how you think or perceive things? What are your hopes and dreams for the present and the future? Do not compare yourself to others because you will always fall short. Instead, try to improve upon yourself day by day! You are a valuable, wonderful person...*unless* you kill puppies or hurt other people *on purpose*.
If that is the case then you are not wonderful. You are awful and you need help.☹

FOR THE REST OF YOU, LOVE YOURSELF! YOU ARE WORTH IT AND DESERVE THE BEST!

- **Date someone long enough and they will show themselves to you:** If you only date someone for a few months, they are still trying to show you their good side. *Analogy: at the car dealership, do they put out ugly cars to sell? Dented, paint peeling, old tires, leaking oil with ripped up seats inside? No. They want the car to be as attractive as possible so they will only put out the best-looking car and wash, wax and shine EVERYTHING on the car.*

The same is true in dating in the sense that when you first begin dating someone they are trying to "sell" themselves to you so they will show you ONLY their best-looking side. Over time, you will be able to see their ugly side and if it is a good person then their ugly side will not be too ugly to deal with.☺ If you are looking for a long-term relationship then be sure to date in person for AT LEAST one year before committing to marriage or a more established relationship, so that you can see the person in all seasons. Online/long distance dating needs even more time!

Especially take note of how they act when they are angry. If you have dated for a while and you have not seen them angry then do something discretely that might anger them--like spill juice on their nice dress or on their car seat--and watch how they react. It might sound mean, but it is very important! It could save you a trip to the emergency room later on! You want to watch how they are with people like waiters at restaurants: if their food is incorrect, do they start cursing or act unreasonably? How do they feel about people of other nationalities and cultures? This can be a sign of their character. See how they are with their family and friends. If a man or woman can call their mother or father bad names, they will not treat you better! Also ask your family and friends what they think about the person you are dating. If you have good and wise family and friends they will let you know if the person you like is a loser or not. You may not see bad qualities because you have "love glasses" on. Be sure to take their opinions seriously!

- **If they treat you badly while you are dating it will only get worse:** This should be the time when they show you their "best looking car"! In an argument if they abuse you **physically** (push, slap, punch, grab, throw something at you or just get into your face in a threatening way) or **emotionally** (call you names or give you the silent treatment) then you should forget about dating this person! If they are *starting* the relationship by showing you the "ugly car"--and if they do ANY of the things I just mentioned above this is the UGLIEST car you could buy--then you do not need them in your life and if you stay with them, you will definitely find yourself in the medical system.

- **You will not change them:** people only TRULY change when they see that there is a problem. They need to change for THEMSELVES and not for you. If they are mean and a bully now, then they will be mean and a bully later too. If they change to please their romantic partner, the change is usually not lasting. People rarely change--or it may take years for them to change so accept them as they are right now or MOVE ON.

Car Analogy: once you drive it away from the car dealership the car begins to age and drive worse...not better! Right? Humans are the same in the sense that once you "buy" or marry/commit to them they typically feel no need <u>to try</u> <u>hard</u> anymore and will relax their behavior! With a car, you have to care for the car to keep it in good condition. As long as you care for the car it will run well even after you buy it. **Humans are a little different because they THINK and cars do not.** Therefore, if a human was only trying to change in order to "sell" himself or herself to you, once you "buy" or marry/commit to them, they may change back to how they were before. That is why it is very important to date a person long enough to see if they are faking or not. Most people will not try to fake ANYTHING past six months, hence my suggestion to date for one year minimum. Faking is too much work and humans can be very lazy.

- **Just broke up? Do not just start a new relationship**! Take time to heal and get over the person before you date someone new. Think about what made that relationship not work--maybe picking the same "bad" type person for you-- and work on fixing yourself. If you do not, then you just carry your bad habits and problems to the next person. This may take anywhere from a few months to a few years. Read self-help books get a counselor or watch YouTube videos.

- **Thinking of getting married?** These concepts can also be applied to long-term relationships for non-married people but being married is both a business and romantic contract and the financial and legal problems that can arise with marriage are very serious so that is why I mention marriage here. All aspects of your health are affected by this person who will share your life so be sure you get premarital counseling and discuss big factors that tend to cause stress and health problems in a relationship such as:

(1) **Children**-do you want them or not? How many and how soon? Have only your own kids and or adopt? How to discipline them? Religious instruction?
(2) **Religion or spirituality**-religion changes a person's <u>behavior</u> so it is *very* important to agree in this area and establish guidelines.
(3) **Finances** -are you a spender or saver? Who or how is the money controlled?

(4) Individual life goals-did you always want to be a singer or painter? Want to go back to school? Make sure you both can walk on life's path together and be prepared to take turns supporting each other while you go after your dreams.

(5) Elderly parents-did you always plan to have your parent(s) living with you when they get old? Because if your spouse or partner did not know this and thought you would put them in a nursing home that can cause a problem

(6) Work-some people do not want their spouse to work (rare!) but if you do want to work you need to discuss this.

(7) Health-you may already have some long-term illness or if you get into a accident how you want to care for yourself or be cared for. It is important to share any current health problem you have with a future legal partner. If your condition gets worse they will have to care for you, so if they did not know that you had any health problems-- maybe you did not know yourself either--then all of a sudden when they go from squeezing your bum (hot) to wiping your bum (not hot) that might be a shock.☹ This is why I also recommend getting blood work and a physical exam before marriage, just in case these items were not already up to date. Again, if your dating partner truly loves you then they will most likely decide to stay with you in spite of illness and then you both can work on building health together but you do not want to surprise them with an illness if it is at all possible.

Match yourself with someone who is equal to you mentally, physically, emotionally and spiritually. Again, you are becoming a team of two!

Analogy: let us use the basketball analogy again. You do not want a player on your team who does not take a shot at the basketball goal because they never think to do it (mentally unequal). You do not want a teammate who <u>chooses </u>*not to train to stay in shape and so they are always tired and a lot slower on the basketball court than you (physically unequal.) Or if every time they take a shot and miss the goal, they throw themselves onto the ground crying and having tantrums then they are emotionally unequal. The idea in a basketball game is to make as many points as possible so pick the BEST teammate from the start! You cannot control how they change with time.*

You should not be identical or too similar though...in fact there is a saying that if *"in a couple the two are too similar, then one of the people is unnecessary!"* ☺ It is good to have differences because that way you help broaden the other person's mind and you can both evolve to be better people. However, it is also not good to be TOO different because then you cannot find a common foundation. What I have seen is best, is for a couple to be in agreement on at LEAST the top three of the seven main factors that affect a relationship and health: children, religion and finances. Age difference is not always a big factor, it depends on the maturity and background of each person however I have seen that typically a difference in age of more than 10-15 years may cause some problems.

RESOURCES: Singles and Dating books/DVDs/CDs by Mark Gungor[65] and Gary Chapman.[66] I have not read their books/seen their videos on singles or dating but I did watch/read their other works that I mentioned before so I am sure anything from these two is worth investigating! They are on point with my real life experiences!

WHY DID YOU GIVE ALL THIS KIND OF ADVICE DR. MEGAN?

You may be thinking that a doctor should only worry about body parts but remember that as doctors we see and hear EVERYTHING that affects a person's health whether it is mental, emotional or physical. We are problem solvers! We are always looking for a way to get to the root of the problem and very often, the origin of the health problem is in a person's self-destructive behavior--drugs, alcohol or hating themselves or someone else. Nevertheless, the root problem can also be in the behavior of someone in their life--parent, sibling, child etc. We must try to find and help them remove the "obstacle to cure" meaning the thing(s) that are keeping them from getting well.

Story: my sister-in-law M is a schoolteacher in a district where many of the kids are from very poor families. Sometimes a kid may come to class and not be able to concentrate because they have not eaten anything since the day before. Therefore, she may give them a snack so that they can feel better and concentrate. Just as teachers see ALL aspects of a student's life--problems at home and school--the same is true of doctors.

In medicine the suffix "ectomy" means to cut out of the body. Therefore, a lumpectomy would be cutting out a lump from somewhere on the body.
Often the person making a patient sick is a close person in their life. Sometimes I want to tell patients that they need a husband-ectomy or a wife-ectomy! Do not worry, I never tell them that though ☺ since I am not in the business of breaking apart families. However, it is true that people can play a strong role **for improving** your health or **against improving** your health so *choose* your inner circle of friends and life partners *wisely*! Sometimes it may be necessary to separate yourself from a person who has only negative effects on you for a period so that you can focus on yourself. Again, as a naturopathic doctor one of the principles I hold to is prevention. Since I see SO many issues arise in a person's health relating to drugs, alcohol, dating/relationships I wanted to mention it here so that perhaps a few of you can avoid these problems! Remember this saying *"A wise man learns from his mistake, but a wiser man learns from the mistakes of others"*. In other words, **do you really need to fly through a windshield to know that a seatbelt is a good thing?!** Let someone else do that!

CHAPTER 10: How liquid fasts help my body clean out trash/detox

24 hours a day, 7 days a week multiplied by however many years you have been alive, your body is CONSTANTLY trying to rid itself of unwanted and harmful chemicals, viruses or bacteria, trash/junk. The body also tries to recover from traumas you have suffered, and to keep you balanced from just the normal aging process. Eventually your body gets overwhelmed and cannot throw out trash anymore.

Analogy: in your house you may have a garage full of junk, boxes under the bed, old magazines/papers in the office, a bunch of old clothes in the closet, random items under the bed and in kitchen cabinets. Likewise, your body has trash and junk stored in fat, muscles and organs that needs to come out because it is making you sick! Repeat: Your body is full of trash!

So a little help from you to clean out this junk is good! Liquid fasts help clean out trash quickly and efficiently! Detoxification is the body breaking down harmful substances via the two main organs of detoxification (Liver and Kidneys) and then removing those bad things from the body by using the four organs of elimination/trash removal: **(1)** Bowels/intestines/colon via pooping, **(2)** Kidneys via peeing, **(3)** Skin via sweating and **(4)** Lungs via breathing out.

Analogy: detoxification is cleaning out all unused/old items from the under the bed, cabinets etc. and placing them in the middle of the living room floor.
Elimination is you actually taking all the old items and placing them outside of the house on the sidewalk for the trash man to pick up!

WHY DOES LIQUID JUICE/TEA FASTING WORK SO GREAT?

Digestion/breaking apart big food you eat takes energy, afterwards you also GET energy from the broken down food. However, juice fasting allows your body to break up a high vitamin and mineral source while using the *least* amount of energy. Liquids are very easy to digest compared to food so the energy you saved from digestion can now be used elsewhere in the body: to fight infection or rebuild an area/body part.

Analogy 1: *would you rather work 3-4 hours standing on your feet and earn only $100 **OR** work 30 minutes seated and earn $1,000? That is literally an example of the difference that juice fasting makes versus eating in saving energy!*
Analogy 2: *what is easier to rip apart a whole book or a piece of paper?*
The idea is to work smarter, <u>not</u> harder! ☺

WHAT TYPES OF LIQUID FASTS ARE THERE?
Two main types **(1)** Water only fasting or **(2)** fasting using vegetable/fruit juice and or herbal teas. Water only fasting should be done under the supervision of a physician, however veggie/fruit/herbal tea fasts can be done while even eating just one small meal a day, perhaps a salad or light meal with veggies and then drinking various combinations of water and fruit and veggie juices and herbal teas.

HOW LONG SHOULD I FAST? HOW INTENSE SHOULD I DO IT?
Beginner: If you have never done one before, you may want to try one day of many different liquids with two tiny meals—breakfast (nuts and fruit) and dinner (beans and green veggies only). Then work your way up to one day a week with only vegetable juice/teas/pure water with no meals.

Intermediate: If you have fasted once or twice previously you could try five days eating only ONE meal a day (breakfast or lunch) and drinking veggie juice/tea*/water throughout the rest of the day. *Non-caffeinated tea.*

Advanced: if you have already fasted extensively, you may decide not to eat at all and only drink healthy liquids for seven to ten days. If doing the advanced level be sure to drink enough liquids or else you will feel hunger! Drink no less than 64 ounces of fluid a day or a 16-ounce drink roughly every 30 minutes or so. If you only drank water, then waiting 15 minutes is usually long enough. If you made a drink with more calories like a vegetable drink or a liquid fruit drink/smoothie then allow about 30 minutes to 1 hour for it to digest before drinking the next drink. Also, please stay close to a bathroom because you will be a peeing machine. ☺

Note: if you do an extended advanced fast with only food and no liquids you MUST slowly re-introduce food! The first day raw foods only; second day cooked vegetables and fruit only and then the third day you can eat regularly or else you will lose any GOOD results you got from fasting and mess up your stomach! ☹

HOW OFTEN SHOULD I FAST?
As often as possible! Depending on your age you have X amount of years of trash to start trying to get rid of. A weekly one day fast is optimal—so maybe a whole day or half day of just veggie drinks, water and herbal teas. A monthly 5-day fast would be the next best. The absolute minimum you should do would be every 3 months a 7 day fast. Again, chemicals from air, water, food, viruses or bacteria and mental/emotional stressors constantly bombard us! Help! ☹ Fast as often as you are able! This is a lifetime thing, **do not think a one-time cleanse will undo YEARS of damage** so make it a part of your lifestyle! Maybe you do not think you have energy to do just a liquid fast. Then pick one day a week or some other period of time where you just eat raw foods or just steamed green veggies, fruit and nuts. It gives your system a "mini" vacation from breaking up heavier foods!

WARNING!! DETOX ALERT! WARNING!

IT IS _HIGHLY DANGEROUS_ to detox with ANY type program or product if you are not BOTH **(1) drinking enough water** for your body weight and **(2) having at least 1 daily bowel movement** that is full and complete meaning you do not feel like there is still poop left in there! **Pooping is the #1 way to get solid trash out of the body and peeing is the #1 way to eliminate liquid trash**. Do not detox improperly! **Analogy:** _you decide to have a yard sale. You clean out your house for the yard sale, removing all junk from under the bed, closets, kitchen cabinets and the garage. However, after having removed all junk from their stored areas, instead of taking it outside of the house immediately, you foolishly block all the exits of the house: so you block the front, back, and garage doors with trash!_

This is dangerous! Why? Because now instead of having an organized house with junk stored away in designated areas like those that we had before, we now have a mess throughout the house! There are a few boxes in the middle of the living room floor for dad to bump into, clothes on the staircase for the kids to trip over and fall down the stairs, as well as old papers scattered on the kitchen floor for mom to slip on! **There is a chaotic mess all over the house, and because you blocked all the doors now you have to climb out of the windows to carry the trash out of the house and onto the lawn for the yard sale!** VERY inefficient and inconvenient, and with health it is dangerous to take out stored toxins/trash and have them moving around in the blood again! Remember, we need water for pooping, peeing and for sweating three of the four main ways we take out trash/waste/toxins from our bodies. **SOLUTION:** drink more water and eat more fiber foods—fiber is like a "broom" that help us sweep out poop!

High fiber foods are:

- **Ground flaxseed**--try a tablespoon a day in food or beverage of choice.
- **Dark green veggies** every day--broccoli, kale, mustard greens, collard greens, spinach
- **Fruits**--especially prunes, apples, and pears but do not peel apple and pear skins that is where the fiber is!
- **Beans, peas and lentils**
- **Nuts and seeds**
- **Whole wheat products**--bran cereals, whole wheat* bread.

*White breads/pastas have REMOVED all fiber!

Remember, get cereals and breads with very low sugar. Sugar is bad.☹

- After *first* <u>adjusting water and fiber/diet,</u> and you still cannot get daily bowel movements then you can order the **ONLY laxative product** I trust which is from Dr. Richard Shulze[4] called **Intestinal #1**. It uses healing herbs to help stimulate/"poke" your bowels to move. It actually helps to retrain bowels and is not habit forming because once your bowels are properly retrained you will not need them any longer. However, how long the training takes depends on your body. For some this takes weeks, months or years. **WARNING:** Other laxative products can offset your body's balance, making those bowel muscles lazy and then you may not be able to poop without the laxatives! **Analogy:** *this is like having a 2-year-old child who can walk but refuses to walk because they always want you to carry them. They just sit on the ground, cry, and will not move if you do not pick them up. Their leg muscles work fine but the child is just lazy. You may be able to carry them all the time at 2 years old, but what about at 5 years old? 10 years old? They are getting bigger and heavier.* This would become a huge problem! We never want ANY part or organ of the body to become lazy because we are giving it some outside product—whether we are using a drug or an herb, INSTEAD we want to help stimulate that area to do its work and operate normally on its own.

MY FAVORITE BLOOD CLEANING JUICE RECIPE!
- 4 ounces/125 mL Carrots
- 2 ounces/ 62 mL Beets and beet greens
- 2 ounces/ 62 mL Wheat grass juice or Cabbage
- 2 ounces/62 mL Water Chestnut

MY FAVORITE FASTING/CLEANSING PRODUCTS!
From Dr. Richard Shulze[4], naturopathic doctor and herbalist. He has 30 day cleanse program(s); 5 day cleanses for **(1)** Bowels/Intestines/Colon **(2)** Liver **(3)** Kidneys, respectively. I HIGHLY recommend his products professionally and continue to use ALL of them myself REGULARLY for healing! **You can do this!**

CHAPTER 11: Doc, help me lose weight! Weight loss formula and tips!

Many people struggle with keeping a healthy weight but there are **four possible reasons why a person will gain weight**:

(1) Medical Conditions-diabetes or low functioning thyroid are a few examples
(2) Medications-weight gain is a common side effect
(3) Stress-especially mental/emotional—causes an increase in Cortisol hormone which can stop your body from fat burning and make you hold onto fat.

BUT **THE MAIN REASON WHY _MOST_ PEOPLE ARE OVERWEIGHT?**
(4) Hypernutrition which is overeating!

DID YOU KNOW?
THAT THE BODY LOVES TO SAVE EXTRA CALORIES LIKE WE SAVE EXTRA MONEY?

Analogy: if someone walked up and offered you $1000, would you say "No thanks, I already earned enough money at work today"? You would not right? You would take the $1000! We cannot ever have too much money! Even if you do not need it for yourself, you can use it for other people or projects. Most of us keep extra money in the bank because money is such a valuable thing to have. The body sees extra calories as "money" to save in the form of FAT for later use as energy.

- So **all extra calories** you eat over the minimum amount of calories that your body actually needs for energy for **TODAY** turn directly to FAT!
- *Even if you are eating <u>healthy foods</u>, once your body has enough calories for the day's energy needs, ALL FOOD turns into FAT! So you should not OVER EAT!*

DID YOU KNOW?
THAT THE BODY DOES NOT LIKE OPEN SPACES?

Analogy: do you remember the cars from the 1940's? You could open the hood and actually crawl into the car to make repairs because there was a lot of open space in there. Now if you open the hood of more recent model cars there is NO extra space under the hood!

- *The body is like the **newer model cars**! While I was in medical school and learning in the anatomy lab, when we would open up a body/cadaver,** there was NO OPEN SPACE ANYWHERE! The body does not like empty spaces because empty spaces are places where infections can happen. If there is not an organ, bone or muscle there the body stores fat.*
- *It will continue to store FAT indefinitely!*

**Funny story: My family came to Arizona to visit me in medical school. While touring the school I showed them the cadaver lab—cadaver faces remained covered out of respect. Upon returning home, my second nephew P—then 13 years old--wrote on his school report about his vacation "I went to visit my aunt Megan and we saw a dead body"! But he did not mention that it was a cadaver and that I was in medical school! I bet the poor school teacher was shocked! But P thought it was really cool. ☺

DID YOU KNOW?
THAT STARVING YOURSELF WILL _STILL_ MAKE THE BODY HOLD ON TO FAT?

Analogy: We will use the same money example as before---but now imagine that you are either unemployed or underemployed. If you are wise you will not spend money if you are not sure when you will earn money again or if you know that you do not have enough money to spend. The body is wise and will not burn calories if it is not sure when you will eat again!
- ***So if you do not eat breakfast*** *then your body begins the day starving—like you going to work but not being sure if they will pay you or not at the end of the work day!*
- ***Yo-yo eating***—*when you eat a lot and then not at all—it makes your body unsure of when you will have food again or when you will get "paid" so it will not burn fat! That is why eating at random times and in random amounts will confuse the body.*

DID YOU KNOW?
THAT EXERCISE IS <u>NOT</u> BURNING OFF ENOUGH EXTRA CALORIES!

Story: Before I became a doctor, one of my jobs was working at a hotel. While I was working there, I gained some extra weight because the hotel used to let us eat free. So I decided to go onto the Weight Watchers weight loss points program, which assigned all foods a certain point value. Based on my weight at that time, the Weight Watchers maximum daily points for me to eat was 20; I went to eat at an Italian restaurant one evening and ordered the fettucine alfredo plate which alone was 24 points! Of course, those were the points for that ONE meal--not counting the garlic bread and salad-and you KNOW that I did not just eat ONE meal that entire day; that was just dinner! I still had to add up the points from breakfast and lunch and so I had eaten 45 points for that day.☹ To make up for it, I decided to go to the gym and exercise, because if you exercised with your heart rate up, you could subtract some of the points from the day. I spent 90 minutes on the treadmill walking/running and sweating to death. By the end, I almost fell off the treadmill! After all that, I only burned 4 points off! ☹

- *Exercising <u>WILL NOT</u> make up for overeating.*
- *Exercising is great for the body, but actually not necessary to lose weight!*
- **The KEY IS NOT TO OVEREAT! IT IS SIMPLE MATH!**

DO PEOPLE EAT WELL IN THIS COUNTRY?

Some do. However, most people eat very poorly in America. We use an acronym to describe the way the average American eats:

The Standard American Diet is "SAD" ☹

- A diet high in: fried foods, fast foods, junk foods
- A diet high in: calories, sugar, salt
- A diet *low* in vitamins, minerals and other necessary nutrients.

WHAT IS THE IDEAL WEIGHT LOSS DIET?

The same guidelines about variety, a colorful plate, more fresh and home cooked, less prepackaged/restaurant/fast food apply. See chapter 8 under Nature's law #3 nutrition. However, these tips will really make a difference for weight loss:

PROTEIN AT EACH MEAL--*helps you feel full—try to get minimum 50 grams of protein a day unless you have a medical condition that restricts protein. Do not eat the same protein type for weeks; eat one or two different types of protein daily or weekly*. Example, if you ate chicken or tofu as your main protein all this week, next week switch to beef, or beans if vegetarian/vegan. The optimal plan is changing protein types daily or weekly. Keep animal food consumption very low and eat more beans, grains and nuts! Remember the formula 70:30. For any meal that has animal based products in it try to make it 70% non-animal foods--like beans, nuts, vegetables, grains--and 30% animal based food--meat, fish, eggs or dairy products. Dairy is anything from a cow like milk, creams, and butter.

Protein rich foods and their relative amounts of protein
Meat sources:
- **Red Meats** (beef, bison, lamb) 3 ounces (oz) average is 25-29 grams (g) of protein.[5]
- **Poultry** (chicken, turkey) 4 oz average is 23-27 g of protein.
- **Fish** (average fish of any type such as salmon) 3 oz is 22 g of protein.

Non meat sources:
- **Beans/lentils** (average for any type) 1 cup is 15-28 g of protein
- **Nuts/seeds** (average for any type) 1 cup is 20 g of protein
- **Grains** (barley, millet and wheat germ are among the highest) 1 cup is 28 g, 25 g, and 17 g respectively.
- **Milk (cow or goat) 1 cup is 8 g** but try to use more goat milk, soy, coconut or almond milk and limit cow's milk because sometimes cow's milk has mucus in it. ☹
- **Egg average size (2 g in the yolk) is 6 g**[6]

HEALTHY FATS AT EACH MEAL--think 1-2 avocados a day--*helps you feel full and provides vitamins and minerals—yes they are fats but they do not make you fat!*

HIGH FIBER FOODS–*help you feel full; feed healthy digestion bacteria; sweep out poop!*
   Foods high in fiber:
- **Ground flaxseed**
- **Dark green veggies every day**--broccoli, kale, mustard greens, collard greens, spinach
- **Fruits**--especially prunes, apples, and pears. Do not peel apple and pear skins, that is where the fiber is!
- **Beans, peas and lentils**
- **Nuts and seeds**
- **Whole wheat products:** bran cereals, whole wheat bread

LOW IN PROCESSED SUGAR--try for 30 grams total or less a day. *Processed/added table sugar is empty calories. Your body takes it in but still feels like it is starving. High sugar containing foods make you actually want to **eat more** leading to weight gain.* **Remember:** your body only makes about 4 g of blood sugar to float around on your highways at any given time…just enough for the energy you need. An average soda has 20 g of sugar! Five times what is necessary! All the extra sugar/calories will turn to what? You guessed it… FAT! ☹ Carefully read ALL packaged food labels for sugar in each SERVING. Remember these other names for sugar: corn syrup/syrup solids, high fructose corn syrup. If it ends in "ol" sorbitol, malitol, xylitol that is also sugar. Definitely avoid artificial sweeteners since these actually "trick" your body because they do not look like normal sugar and so you really eat more of these than you want to because they are wearing a "mask/disguise" that says to your body "I am not sugar" and then you really gain weight! It is always better to use regular table sugar than something fake made in a laboratory somewhere!

LOW IN SALT *(1500 mg/day)*--highly salty foods make your body hold onto water leading to an overall weight gain. Remember, if you are cooking most of your food you will not over salt. *Consult your physician if you are on a salt restriction diet.*

WHAT IS THE SECRET WEIGHT LOSS FORMULA??
W2H2. The W2 stands for <u>what</u> and <u>when</u> you eat, and the H2 stands for <u>how much</u> and <u>how often</u> you eat. Ok, so technically, it is not a secret because you have seen this formula earlier in chapter 8 under the nutrition section but there is some extra information here:

MAIN TIPS

- **Watch WHAT you eat**—Avoid S.A.D. Foods: fast food/fried food/junk food/vending machine foods. Eat these twice a week MAXIMUM and in very small quantities. Do not have unhealthy food available in the cupboards at home it will only be a temptation. *It is easier to take and eat a bag of chips from the cabinet at midnight then it is to have to get dressed and go OUT and buy a bag of chips at midnight.* ☺ Plan your meals ahead. If you do not want to cook daily/hate to cook then pick one or two days to cook for the entire week. *Have designated eating out days—usually one weekend meal is best.* Always carry healthy snacks--nuts with raisins or even raw carrots/celery sticks--so you do not have to stop and buy unhealthy food just because you got caught out somewhere and now you are starving.
    - **Eat filling foods**--at each meal have protein, a healthy fat and sufficient fiber
    - **Eat crunchy foods**--there is a link between having **chewed** a lot and the feeling fullness. The more time spent chewing food, the brain interprets that as having eaten a lot of food and lowers the "I'm hungry eat more" hormone called Ghrelin. ***Example: we can eat a plate of spaghetti (soft) but NOT a plate of raw carrots (hard).*** *Your jaw will start hurting by the third carrot so then you stop eating!*
    - **Avoid empty and hidden calories**--ESPECIALLY TABLE SUGAR! Beware of salad dressings and beverages--obviously soda, but also coffee and FRUIT JUICES; make water your main drink!
    - **Stay hydrated**--the minimum to drink refers to water alone with nothing added into it! T*ea or lemonade does not count. They are no longer water!* ☹ Drink half your body weight in ounces*unless you have a water restriction illness. So if you weigh 200 pounds drink 100 ounces daily. Drink more if you live/work in a hot environment or exercise. *Dehydration is often mistaken for hunger because hunger and thirst travel on the same "road/nerve" from Stomach city back up to Brain city and sometimes the Brain can get confused. If you are not sure if you are truly hungry or not, first drink 16 oz of water wait 20 minutes and if you are still hungry/your stomach is actually growling then that is true hunger! EAT!*

- **Watch WHEN you eat**--*Analogy: when is your household busiest and moving fastest? Probably in the morning right? You wake up early to run out the door to work and get the kids off to school. Then when everyone returns in the evening the pace is much slower; you sit in front of the TV, and do school work etc. Your body does the same thing. We call this metabolism. It is usually fastest first thing in the morning. Early in the day is when you burn more calories compared to later in the day when metabolism is slower. So DO NOT eat heavy meals with a lot of food or even harder to digest foods like proteins late in the evening when your body is already slowing down! Eat heavier meals at breakfast and lunch, and then lighter meals at dinner, unless you work overnight and then your meal right before work should be the heaviest. That way you can burn off some fat when you are moving around!*
    - **Eat with a routine**--at approximately the same times daily. The body likes to know when food is coming. Eat 2-3 well-spaced meals a day--it helps avoid snacking. ***Analogy***: *do you remember the paycheck example? Sporadic eating is like working one day and then not working the next day. You do not really know how much money you will make to pay your monthly bills. Likewise, the body will not know whether to hold onto or to burn calories because your eating is not regular so it will likely hold onto calories/fat.*
    - **Stop eating 3 hours prior to bedtime**—*your stomach and intestines have worked hard ALL day and deserve to start winding down to go to bed. If you make them work at bedtime it just makes them mad and they will not digest properly. You probably will not sleep well which will make you tired (and mean) in the morning. Studies have shown that poor sleep can lead to overeating!* ☹☹

- **Watch HOW MUCH you eat**--do not eat in excess of daily needs! This depends on your occupation and physical activity level but the average for women is around 1800 calories/day and for men 2400 calories/day. However, do not starve yourself either. Trick your brain by using your eyes! Use smaller sized plates and fill it completely with food so that your brain feels as if you have eaten a lot versus using a larger size plate that holds less food and your brain deciding that maybe you should eat more because the plate is so big.

- **Watch HOW OFTEN you eat**--if you have a desk job, you likely can just eat two well-spaced meals a day with a light snack at dinner. If you work construction or another physically demanding job, you may need to eat three meals a day. No one should need to eat more than three meals a day unless you are seriously an Olympic athlete or something! I do not mean in ping pong, I mean in track and field or gymnastics! Nothing against ping-pong. ☺
- **Avoid eating and watching TV**--Studies have shown we eat more when we watch TV because of all the food commercials! Seriously, do an experiment and count how many commercials are about FOOD on TV. The only thing more advertised than food commercials are drug/medicine commercials. Hmmm. Makes you wonder! They do this at the movie theatre too with the popcorn and soda commercials before the movie starts! Measure your meal BEFORE you sit down to watch TV—meaning do not take an entire bag of chips to the TV, take out 15 chips so that you do not overeat!

Notes:
(1) take small bites. Do not have your cheeks extend out like a chipmunk. Chipmunk cheeks are cute on chipmunks...not on humans. ☹ Bite enough food to keep it in the middle of your mouth. If you take small bites, then you can chew the food really well. The more you chew the less you eat. A *mouth full of food* makes you chew less and swallow **more** food *faster*. ☹

(2) take a small bite and then put the sandwich/slice/bag/fork/spoon down. **Example:** when you take a bite of a sandwich and leave the sandwich directly in front of your mouth, it makes you chew faster because your eyes see that there is more food close to your mouth! When you take a bite and lower the food and or utensil back onto the plate, you can concentrate on carefully chewing the food. You will chew more and eat less! Remember to chew food until it is almost liquid! No big chunks of food should go down to Stomach city. There are no teeth in there! Big pieces of food in Stomach city will lead to big health problems.☹ This will take practice but you can do this! The only object to keep close to your mouth so that you can consume it quickly and in large quantities is a WATER BOTTLE. Do not sip water! Drink at least 2-3 cups in one sitting. Preferably away from meals.

(3) many people feel the need to "clean" their plates or not leave food behind because it is wasteful. Again, if you pick a *small* plate—such as a bread plate--you will not leave food behind. If you are at a restaurant ask them to put half of your food into the "to go" container. If you do not want to eat the restaurant food later then leave it behind! There is no reason to overeat just because your parents told you that you should not leave food on the plate. Which is smarter? Caring for your health or wasting money on doctors and hospitals? Additionally, if someone buys you a food that you know is very harmful to your health, you do not have to eat it only to satisfy them or not have them waste their money! Again, which is more important? To make them feel good and so you eat the entire pie that is FULL of sugar...or to eat a slice and then throw the rest of the pie away? You do not have to tell them that you threw it away but you DO need to care for your health! A pie costs $10. A hospital stay or surgery will be thousands. Even I can do that math.

LAST WEIGHT LOSS TIPS:
Most people are overweight because they OVER EAT! Often people will tell me, Doc, I have to eat a lot because I am hungry! Remember these things:
(1) That you may actually be THIRSTY and not hungry
(2) Make sure you are not eating just because other people around you are eating or because you are bored
(3) Some people over eat because of emotional states of being--like when they are sad, angry, stressed or want to have control over some part of their life
(4) You may be overeating because you have poor sleeping habits
(5) Your body may be telling you to eat because you are not giving it what it needs so it keeps asking you for it!

Analogy: I am sure that you have been in a toy store and seen this with someone else's kids or maybe even lived this experience with your own kids. The child asks for a specific toy saying "Mom/Dad can I have a doll/toy truck please? You ignore them. They become quiet. Then they ask again later on...MOM... Maybe you try to distract them by letting them push the cart while you are still shopping. They may play with it for a second but then they come back again asking for the doll/toy truck. MOM! DAD! Can I have a doll/toy truck? They will keep on asking until you buy it for them or until you tell them that you WILL NOT buy it and you leave the store. If you did not buy the toy they will be upset.

For MOST people the fifth reason is very common. Your body is asking you for food that has NUTRITION/something good like vitamins, minerals or for more of a certain type of food maybe, like healthy fat or protein. However, you are not giving your body what it is asking for. You ignore it completely or you give it something different from what your body wants like too much sugar, salt or junk. Hence, your brain keeps telling you to EAT hoping that FINALLY you will give it what it wants! Does this make sense? So once you learn the portions to eat, and the food types to mix together, you will get the vitamins, minerals, carbohydrates, protein and healthy fat that you need, and you will see how LITTLE amount of food you actually need to eat when the meal is well balanced!
Remember, **you can do this!**

WEIGHT LOSS AND HEALTHY MEAL RESOURCES

If you want to lose weight, or simply hate cooking and grocery shopping as I do and you want healthy meal choices I have some help for you! There are two ways to eat well. Either you can order fresh healthy meals or you can have someone prepare them for you! The resources below are local in Atlanta; however look for a similar resource in your state or country!

(1) FRESH N FIT CUISINE.[71] This is a _**fantastic**_ service! You can have healthy, local, seasonal foods delivered to your door or pick them up from a nearby pickup station! They ship within Georgia, Alabama and even parts of Florida, the Carolinas and Tennessee! The meal plans vary and include meat, vegetarian, Gluten free, low carb and Paleo diets! You can even customize a meal plan! A registered dietician formulates all meals to ensure adequate calories. A chef prepares the meals in a state of the art United States Department of Agriculture approved kitchen!

I know the president of the company, Mr. Elston Collins, personally and he shares the same passion about health as I do! I have visited the kitchen and facilities and even have personal experience with the food! You can order the meals incrementally—meaning you can order only breakfast or dinner for a week or all three meals for a month or forever! There is no contract! The BEST part is that each meal is only $7.50! Even if you buy fast food, you would spend approximately half that amount for _TRASH_! You would pay more than $7.50 to eat _MEDIOCRE_ food at a typical sit-in restaurant, whereas with this meal you are eating healthily! You spend little to no effort! My mother's pickup station was one mile from her house! No dishes! ☺

(2) PLAN TO PLATE.[72] Another _**fantastic**_ service! If you hate grocery shopping-as I do-they will plan your meal AND do the grocery shopping! Perhaps you do not hate cooking-as I do-but you hate cutting meat and washing vegetables. They will cut, wash and prepare the ingredients so that YOU can cook them, as you would like! Maybe you hate ALL aspects of cooking-like me, although I make myself do it now-they will prepare fully cooked meals for you, even in your home!

I also happen to be acquainted with the owner Ms. Ashli Price. She has a true zeal and passion for healthy, beautiful food!

Both Fresh N Fit cuisine[71] and Plan to Plate[72] are great short-term or long-term options! Short-term examples would be if you expect to have a busy workweek or are moving. Long-term examples would be if you are busy planning a wedding, or if you want to lose weight.

(3) PROFESSIONAL HELP. If you would like to work with a **naturopathic doctor** who **specializes in weight loss** and is passionate about it then I HIGHLY recommend **Dr. Firlande Volcy!** [50] She is very fun and motivating! She could help a seal lose weight with her effective programs! Remember, seals have NOTHING but body fat! Therefore, you are already better off than a seal! However, please only contact her if you are SERIOUS AND PREPARED TO TAKE ACTION to lose weight. **She does not like to work with lazy people or those who make excuses**. I do not blame her. Neither do I.☹ **It is a waste of your time and money and a waste of our time and energy.** It is ok to be realistic and not make many changes at once. If you decide to change only one thing, then at least try to be serious at 100% about that one change! We will accept 99.9% serious people too.☺

CHAPTER 12: Natural medicine is not outdated/hocus pocus! Drugs do not heal!

WHAT ARE THE PROBLEMS WITH ONLY USING PHARMACEUTICAL DRUGS AND SURGERY?

I often receive this question, and there is definitely a time for over the counter/prescription medications and surgery, but I believe that they are 90% OVER USED! I am not against ALL prescribed pharmaceutical/over the counter drug use and ALL surgeries ALL of the time, ***however I AM against MOST pharmaceutical drug use and MOST surgeries, <u>MOST OF THE TIME</u>!***

SURGERY

If you have an IMMEDIATE life threatening condition/issue: such as you are bleeding from a gunshot wound, have experienced some sort of trauma--fallen from a significant height, have a knife sticking out of your hand, or have been in a car accident and you have serious physical injury--then OF COURSE surgery is warranted! Or if a baby is born without a top lip/cleft palate and cannot even eat because of it then surgery is great! But if you have been ***<u>allowed to schedule</u> your surgery instead of being told that you have to have surgery RIGHT NOW or else you will die*—then you *definitely do not need surgery right this second*** and chances are you have time to reflect on how you got outside of Nature's 9 and how you can now choose to get back in balance so that you can strive to keep your natural body parts!

*In this country if your life is truly in danger, a hospital will all but force you into the operating room, if for nothing else so as not to risk a lawsuit from you or your family later! Also in the U.S. we do not let people die because of a lack of money if it is truly an emergency...so even if the person does not have insurance or the money to pay for the surgery the hospital will perform surgery immediately if it is truly life or death. So again, if your surgery can be **scheduled** a few days, weeks or months from now, you are not dying!* These are the ***most common U.S. surgeries*** in no particular order: ***(1)*** *Heart surgeries--bypass, angioplasty/stent or pacemaker; **(2)** Cesarean section **(3)** Hysterectomy **(4)** Back surgery **(5)** Gall bladder removal **(6)** Knee/hip replacement surgery **(7)** Digestive system surgeries--gastric bypass, surgery for heartburn or for Irritable Bowel Syndrome.* One of the top three most common surgeries performed in the U.S. is the hysterectomy, where the uterus/baby hotel is removed from a woman—usually because of her having heavy bleeding or very painful periods/menstrual cycles.

In 2007, the CNN news channel released an article based on a 2005 study about the high amount of unnecessary hysterectomies done in the U.S. They compared the rates of hysterectomies to two other countries. Hysterectomies are performed TWICE as much on American women than on women from the country of England and performed FOUR times more often on American women than on women from the country of Sweden![7] In the article, a gynecological surgeon from an extremely prestigious hospital in New York called Weil-Cornell Medical Center was quoted saying that of the over 600,000 hysterectomies performed every year in the U.S. that 76-85% may be unnecessary! *Gasp!* **This is a GYNECOLOGICAL SURGEON saying this!** That is his day job folks! ***Analogy:*** *That is like a mechanic telling you that 76-85% of the work that he will do on your car, and charge you **A LOT** of money for, is probably unnecessary! On top of that, after he finishes the work on your car, your car will probably drive WORSE than it did before!*

Would you accept that from your mechanic? NO! You would take your car elsewhere and get a second/third opinion from other mechanics or you would let your cousin Frank work on it! Why do you accept it from the healthcare system? Elsewhere in the article, another medical doctor who is a clinical professor of gynecology at the University of California at Los Angeles and the author of the 2005 study on unnecessary hysterectomies in the U.S. stated that the hysterectomy should be **_considered_** mainly if a woman has <u>uterine cancer</u> but that in actuality 90% of hysterectomies performed in the U.S. were performed for *reasons other* than to treat women with uterine cancer![7] Surgery is not without risk since one never knows how an individual will react to the anesthesia and other procedures required for surgery. Even a routine/commonly performed surgery could be deadly for you based on how your individual body reacts! This is why a person can walk into a clinic or hospital for knee replacement surgery and die instead! Additionally, after surgery scar tissue will form in that site blocking some function and therefore that area will no longer work as well as it should.

Why do we love to cut so much in America? Two reasons I believe (1) the conventional medical system does not properly warn the patient about the risk versus benefit of surgery. At times even the doctors themselves are not educated enough to recognize when a surgery is truly necessary or not and often do not even truly understand the function of the organ/part they want to remove. ***(2) but also YOU the patient do not try to look for other solutions, or get second opinions and you just want what you think will be a "quick fix" to a problem,*** *even if you were first advised by your doctors to make lifestyle changes!* ☹

I sincerely believe that if we did not have anesthesia to use during surgery, and then pain medications to use AFTER surgery--medications that either put us to sleep or cover up/eliminate pain thereby tricking us into minimizing the serious nature of surgery—if we could FEEL surgery—then we would truly understand how traumatic it is to the body! Then MOST of us would think TWICE before we so quickly decide to undergo what <u>most of the time</u> is an unnecessary surgery!

With any surgery, you must consider the benefit of the surgery versus the risk/cost. During surgery, there is risk of bleeding, damage to organs, and bad reactions to anesthesia and death. ☹ After surgery cost would be infection, pain and suffering, scarring, long term or lifelong loss of a function and the recovery time required to take off from work/school or activities.
BEFORE UNDERGOING ANY SURGERY GET A 2nd, 3rd and 4th opinion!

WHY MOST DRUGS ARE AWFUL AND DO NOT HEAL!

Drugs are EXTREMELY overused and would likely not be necessary AT ALL if we would just get back in tune with Nature's 9! For example, if you are often overeating greasy fried foods—that is very likely to make your blood pressure be high because it makes your blood be sticky and greasy too--which makes it harder for Heart city to pump around and so it increases blood pressure. Increasing BP medication is not the answer because it can only do so much since you are constantly eating poorly. **Analogy:** *That is like putting a grown man on one side of a see-saw and a 3 year old boy on the other side of the see-saw. The grown man will always have his legs on the ground and the 3 year old boy will always be suspended in the air. Taking medications is like expecting the 3 year old boy to be able to lift the grown man up off the ground! The child is not heavy enough to counteract the size of the man!* Likewise, no amount of medication—no matter WHAT ILLNESS/DISEASE it is prescribed for, or at what dose, will be able to counteract being out of tune with Nature's 9 Health Laws. There are **two main reasons** why most pharmaceutical drugs (prescribed or over the counter) are harmful and do not heal:

(1) Remember, most pharmaceutical medications go against the body's natural methods of healing—*Analogy: You are familiar with a fire alarm right? Its purpose is to make a loud sound so that you know that there is a potential danger for fire in your home. There is either smoke somewhere, or an actual fire. It is VERY rare that a fire alarm will sound because of malfunction/without smoke or fire, so for the most part we can trust the alarm when it goes off. One night, the fire alarm wakes you up in the middle of the night. You are very angry about the alarm and instead of going to check for smoke or fire; you simply turn off the fire alarm and go back to bed. Now you are asleep with NO alarm to warn you of potential danger! This is EXTREMELY dangerous! Fire fighters estimate that it only takes 2 minutes for a home fire to become life threatening. The smoke is what kills people three times more than the flames kill people. It takes 5 minutes for the flames to engulf the average size house/apartment after a small fire has started. This is because of the* *existence of numerous flame accelerants found in modern homes!*[8] *That is why a smoke alarm is so important!*

A fever is the body's way of sounding an alarm and letting us know there is an infection or something else in the body that we need to investigate. However, what do most of us do? We take an anti-fever medication to lower the fever; the illness remains, but now we are unaware of it! Most of us begin turning off body alarms in childhood. By the time we reach senior citizen age the body was forced FOR YEARS to "turn off its fire alarm/fever" so that it will no longer produce a fever EVEN IF A PERSON DOES HAVE AN INFECTION! Why not? Because making a fever takes the body energy, but if we use medications that constantly turn off the body's alarm/fever, the body will not continue to waste energy to make an alarm/fever. ***Analogy:*** *how long would you get up early to go to work only for them to keep sending you home once you arrive at work, telling you that they do not need you to work that day?* Older people will often go to the hospital with an infection, but because the body no longer creates a fever/alarm to signal physicians of an infection or other problem, the senior may not receive the proper treatment!

In naturopathic medicine we would actually use certain methods that will ENHANCE the body's signal/fever/alarm and then monitor the body, instead of just turning off the body's wise signal/alarm.*When someone has a fever, it is wise to consult a healthcare professional that understands that this is the body's sign of a problem and will work with that person to enhance how their body responds. High fevers can be potentially very dangerous therefore always consult a medical professional.*

BOOK ALERT: Woo Hoo! Three fourths of the way through the book! ☺

(2) Remember most pharmaceutical medications mask/hide a symptom in one area while damaging other organs—which is what causes side effects—the body must break down most pharmaceutical drugs. The main organ doing this job is the liver, however the second organ that will help are the kidneys. ***Remember:*** *You can think of these organs as being like metal detectors in an airport, if these two organs see any harmful things coming into the body, they will try to get rid of them—whether it is a drug, food, drink or strange chemical. Since most prescribed medications are seen as harmful by the liver, it would normally get rid of them. Essentially the "metal detector will beep" and then the liver will grab that drug and remove it from the body before it can harm you...just like if they found a gun in your bag at the airport! However, since drug manufacturers know that the liver works this way, they make drugs that have a much higher dose than what would normally be needed so that they can OVERWHELM the liver so that some of the* medication can escape and get into your body. Remember that we call this process of using very high doses to overwhelm the liver the **first pass effect**.

So with the airport example, you have SO many guns hidden all over--in your hand bag, suitcase and one inside of your hat--that the metal detectors get overwhelmed by how many guns there are and miss a few of them, allowing you to carry a gun onto the plane! The bad thing about having these higher doses is that yes, it will hide the symptom that the drug was originally prescribed for, but the medication is making the liver (and often kidneys) work MUCH harder to break apart the drug, which is slowly weakening and destroying both of them! In the **example of the fever** earlier, you decide to take an anti-fever medication. Not only does the anti-fever medication turn off your body's natural fire alarm/fever, but also it makes your liver and kidneys work harder. This damages them, and by damaging them, you cause side effects: high cholesterol or even high blood pressure. Why? Because Liver city is in charge of making and breaking down cholesterol. Kidney city plays a big role in keeping blood pressure in range—along with the heart! See why this is SUPER unhealthy!

Another drug analogy: *Let us say that you burned your RIGHT hand on a hot pot. You cover the right hand with a bandage. This bandage is only covering the burn; there is NO burn ointment on it. Recall that most medications only cover symptoms—such as pain—but do NOT address the cause of the problem and therefore are NOT healing you. Now, imagine that every time you had to change the bandage on your RIGHT hand, just after you changed it, you smashed your LEFT hand with a hammer! Ouch! If you have to change the bandage once every few days, imagine how this will destroy your LEFT hand! Most of us do not take medications every few days; we take them DAILY multiple times a day!* This hammer example is very similar to what happens when we take medications that only cover a symptom in one area (right hand) while doing NOTHING to heal the initial problem, and then INSTEAD harm ANOTHER area of the body (left hand). **You are paying a lot of money for these harmful medications!** ☹
I do not know about you, but that sounds like a bad deal to me.

Now, since you are taking a medication that is harming your body/stopping a normal function, this is often where side effects come in, and sometimes if side effects are bad enough, you will stop taking the medication on your own. However, the liver and kidneys are strong organs. You can destroy them without having a sign/symptom or any side effects until they are very damaged! Because you do not feel anything, or if you only feel a slight headache, or a little upset stomach you keep taking these harmful drugs!

Since most of you do not know where the liver or kidneys are in the body or what their jobs are, you do not think about how medications harm them. But since you DO understand the value of going through life without a hand--*stop right now and think about everything you use your hands for from the moment you get up, until you go to bed.........You use your hands for **EVERYEVERYTHING** right?* Once you smash that left hand with a hammer long enough, you can kiss that hand good bye! Understanding the function as well as the necessity of a hand, then you would not do anything to harm the hand. You would not let anyone smash your hand with a hammer! Not even once! Well your liver and kidneys EACH do *at least 4 times* the amount of things your hand can do! **You CAN live without hands, YOU CAN NOT LIVE WITHOUT A LIVER OR WITHOUT KIDNEYS!** *You will die! You cannot live a good life when either of them does not work well!* **You exist you do not LIVE!** ☹

*By the way here is one **website** that you can use to **look up the potential side effects of a medicine** you have been prescribed **www.rxlist.com.** Many of the side effects are listed in plain English but a few of them are in medical terminology.* **It is true that not ALL people get the same side effects, but any side effect listed means that SOME ONE got that side effect.** ☹

WHERE DO MEDICATIONS COME FROM ANYWAY?
In the United States some are made from zero in a laboratory, others from animal, marine or microbial (bacteria, fungi) sources.[9] But did you know that 70% are made from plants? [10] *Gasp!* Close your mouth now. Yes indeed, 90 of 121 of the most common US medications are made from plants or plant parts: tree bark, flowers, leaves, fruits, roots.[11] Did you know that 47% of anti-cancer drugs come from natural products or natural product mimics?[12]

WHY DO WE USE SO MANY PRESCRIBED MEDICATIONS IN THE U.S?
Because we cannot sell plants and make tons of money! Plants belong to the world, and we cannot patent or own a plant. However, in the 1800's scientists discovered they could isolate a part of a plant to form a drug from it---that is when the pharmaceutical drug industry began in the U.S. Now the pharmaceutical companies can say that WE made this drug with our knowledge and resources so now we will charge you an exorbitant amount of money for our drug!
They cannot charge you $2000 for a flower, because flowers belong to the Earth, which belongs to all of us, but they can charge you $2000 for a cancer medication that they developed from a part of a flower!

U.S. STATISTICS ON HEALTH AND THE COST OF DRUG USE

- The U.S. spent $234 billion on prescription medications in 2008, TWICE the amount spent in 1999. [13]
- The average amount spent on drugs a year per person is $985.[14]
- The U.S. is ranked #1 in how much they <u>spend</u> on healthcare *(bad)*, but in terms of *actual health* ranks #26 out of 34 compared to other rich/developed countries.[15] *(very bad!)*

WHAT DO THESE STATISTICS MEAN?

Every year we are spending ALOT (and more and more) of our hard earned money on medications that are not helping us to heal, and INSTEAD we are getting sicker and sicker! In fact, we are one of the SICKEST countries, even though we are in the top 10 of the most developed/richest countries!

WHAT DOES THE REST OF THE WORLD USE AS MEDICINE?

Did you know that according to the World Health Organization (WHO) 80% of the REST of the world still uses traditional/natural medicines as the **only** or primary form of medicine![16]

So it looks like most of the world is healthier than Americans are and they are using mainly plants so it makes you think doesn't it? **You can do this!**

CHAPTER 13: The 3 drugs that I HATE the most because they hurt you!

It is NO secret that I am not a fan of medications (prescribed or over the counter) and again, that is primarily because they stop your body from doing what it needs to do to naturally to heal itself. They only mask symptoms and do not actually heal anything. They cause extra problems somewhere else! Later on you will read how many medications deplete/pull out vitamins and minerals that you need for basic functioning. The drugs pull out these items from Digestion city, just as a leech would be sucking your blood! *However, even leeches can be used medically to help bring about healing in certain situations, so leeches are STILL better than most of these drugs in my opinion!* ☺ Of the many medications that exist out there, these three are the WORST because of how they work against your body: Antibiotics, Steroids and Antacids.

ANTIBIOTICS

Most antibiotics are medications which kill or slow down the growth of **bacteria only, not viruses**. The discovery of potent antibiotic drugs during this century is recognized as the greatest single advance in the treatment of hundreds of diseases. The speed with which these drugs can reverse certain infections has created the impression of a "miracle drug" in the public mind; such that today most patients with contagious illnesses expect an antibiotic prescription. Naturopathic doctors try to avoid the use of antibiotics whenever possible. This reluctance lies in our recognition that infections can occur **only** when the body is in a <u>vulnerable or weak </u>state. Even during epidemic illnesses, many people exposed to the bacteria or viruses do not get the disease. But these same individuals may become sick with the same illness at another time in their lives when their immune system/internal police are weak.

Three reasons to avoid antibiotics: overuse resistance, nonspecific killers and side effects!

First many bacteria are only susceptible to certain antibiotics. Use of a broad-spectrum antibiotic (it kills many different bacteria) without performing laboratory culture--identifying the actual bacteria by growing it--and sensitivity tests can lead to treatment failure. **Example:** you have a cough with phlegm. They take a sample from the back of your throat of the phlegm/mucus you coughed up. To try to investigate what type of "bug" it is, we need to grow the sample on a special disk in order to figure out if it is a virus, bacterium or fungus and that usually takes a few DAYS! You do not want to wait for days right? You need help now! Because the doctor is "betting or guessing" that it is *probably* a bacterium and you are screaming at the doctor that you need a medication RIGHT NOW…

Ok, maybe you are not screaming but you are very unhappy. You are prescribed an antibiotic which you go home and take immediately for 7 to 10 days. But what if the "bug" making you sick is not actually a bacterium but a virus or a fungus? Well that means that the antibiotic that you just took will not even kill them because most antibiotics only work against BACTERIA!

Analogy: *that is like if we had a poison that will only kill cockroaches but we try to use it anyway on a spider. The spider will just laugh at you and keep on walking! Can spiders laugh??* Maybe it <u>was</u> actually a bacterium, but one that does not die with the *kind* of antibiotic your doctor just prescribed you. The doctor was guessing after all. Therefore, the antibiotic just HURTS the bacterium a little bit. That bacterium actually needed another type of antibiotic to *KILL* him. So your mean bacterium limps away from you, but now he knows how to protect himself against YOU (and the doctor) even better in the future. In this way, many bacteria mutate/change themselves and become immune/protected against antibiotics, thus requiring stronger and stronger antibiotics to kill the bacteria. These drug-resistant strains of bacteria have developed because of the widespread overuse of antibiotics, and are becoming a major threat because if we continue at this rate, when we do want to use an antibiotic it will not work AT ALL against ANY bacteria!

Analogy: *if we made a cockroach spray that killed <u>black</u> cockroaches but then we overused this spray—like sprayed it around the house even when we did not see any black cockroaches, eventually the black cockroaches may start to get accustomed to the overused spray. They will begin to change their DNA and mutate to become <u>brown</u> cockroaches and then the original black cockroach spray will not work against them anymore!*

Second, antibiotics are nonspecific killers, meaning they just look for bacteria to kill. When the antibiotic finds bacteria, it will kill the "bad" bacteria making you sick, but it will ALSO kill your "good" bacteria in Digestion city that are actually trying to help you fight the infection! **Analogy:** *Imagine a burglar breaks into your home and takes your family hostage, but you manage to escape outside and call the police. The first police car comes to your house and a few of them rush inside while you wait outside, but from the looks of things, they are not having a lot of luck stopping the burglar inside. A second police car arrives outside and they decide to just throw a bomb into the house—with no warning—even though the first police that arrived AND your family are still inside with the burglar! The second police want to throw a bomb in there just so they can hurry up and finish with the situation quickly.*

Do you see the problem with that? Not only do they risk hurting the first police that ran inside (who are trying to HELP you) but also they may blow up your family members too because bombs destroy anything within their blow up radius! Likewise, antibiotics do not distinguish between your internal police/immune system bacteria that are fighting to get you healthy again or your family members/digestion bacteria you need for basic good health! **On top of all that, if the antibiotic was not specific to the bacterium making you sick, then you do not even hurt the burglar AT ALL!!** He escapes from the back window, and watches as your family members and the first police blow up! He laughs and then runs away to burglarize another house! ☹

A **third** reason I hate them is that antibiotics often cause various side effects including:
- Rashes, hives, or other allergic reactions
- Stomach pain, cramps, diarrhea, vomiting-slows or messes up digestion and use of vitamins and nutrients. *Noooo!!!! Dr. Megan is screaming because we are blowing up her specialty area...also known as the Washington D.C. of you! Teardrop, sigh, sadness!* ☹
- Kidney or liver damage
- Phlebitis/inflammation of the blood vessels
- Overgrowth of Candida and other yeast in the vagina--women will often get yeast infections post antibiotic use and overgrowth in the intestines (can lead to brain fog and fatigue)

So you see? Antibiotics do not strengthen the patient's body; they only kill bacteria, thus failing to correct the underlying weakness that allowed the infection to occur in the first place. Many patients become long-term unhealthy or get frequent or repeated infections--cold/flu/ear/digestion infections etc. after overuse of antibiotics, because as we already said, they kill healthy bacteria that are part of your immune system, as well as the unhealthy bacteria that may be causing illness. Medical research has even shown that recovery from some infections is more complete if antibiotic drugs are not used early in the course of the illness because allowing the police/immune system to fight the illness is beneficial. In general, a healthy immune system will kill bad bacteria, viruses or fungi before a long-term illness develops. Remember, it is not a problem to catch a cold/flu/other infection once or twice a year. It strengthens the immune system. If you are sick more often than that, your immunity is too low. Sadly, we do not give nature a chance and instead use/misuse antibiotics. A quote from a recent article from the Centers for Disease Control (CDC): "studies estimate that 30-50% of antibiotics prescribed in hospitals are unnecessary or inappropriate".[17] Those statistics are in hospitals--we have not even discussed the statistics for over prescribing antibiotics at the doctor's office or urgent care!

What should I do if I get an infection?

Dr. Megan, are you saying NEVER to use antibiotics and to let a raging infection go untreated? No! See, there you readers go again, putting words into my mouth! ☹ Unless you are trained in how to handle an infection with natural means--*which by the way, natural medicines and combined therapies can treat pretty much ANY infection even serious ones*--then of course you cannot just let an infection go unchecked!

But what I am saying, is **(1)** do not run to your doctor ***demanding*** an antibiotic at the first sign of illness for you or your child--without having first identified what bug is making you/them sick **(2)** remember if you got sick in the first place, then you must get back in tune with Nature's 9 to get well. With any short-term illness (cold/flu/upset stomach): avoid eating unless you are actually hungry. If you are hungry, then eat NO SUGAR, NO BREAD, NO MEAT, NO RICE, NO PASTA, NO CEREALS, NO JUICE and NO DAIRY while you are sick and even *up until two days after your symptoms go away.* Eat beans, soup, nuts and green vegetables. Meat and dairy take a lot of energy to digest. They take fighting bugs/police energy away and that energy is used towards digestion energy instead. ☹ We do not want to waste energy on digestion when we have evil bugs to fight! Additionally, carbohydrate foods such as those listed above, are energy sources for the bad bacteria, virus or fungi. Therefore, you give them energy to fight AGAINST you! Drink plenty of **plain** water (NO other beverages unless it is non-caffeinated fresh herbal tea) and most importantly, rest and try to get fresh air and sunshine and you should be back on your feet soon! If you are not better after this, it means your immune system is already SUPER weak! **(3)** Try to have a friendly neighborhood naturopathic doctor on speed dial that you can go and see in a pinch, which IS TRAINED to offer better options! ☺

STEROIDS

Are typically used to **(1)** decrease short-term or long-term inflammation and **(2)** to suppress the immune system. Cream or lotion based steroid medications are often used on skin infections. Steroids can be used inside the body also: as an injection into joints like for knee and back/spine problems or as oral medications for those with autoimmune diseases. Autoimmune diseases are those in which the body becomes confused and attacks itself instead of attacking a bad object that is not part of the body. Diseases like Multiple Sclerosis, Lupus, Rheumatoid Arthritis and Diabetes Type 1. **Analogy:** *Autoimmune disease is like if a police officer runs into a bank robbery and shoots the bank robber, but then gets confused and shoots the bank teller, a person in line who just came to get some money and even shoots a second police officer who ran inside to help him!*

These medications are also VERY strong and when used at very specific and limited times can be very helpful and lifesaving! However, like most medications often they are used improperly or are overused and as a result destroy the body instead of helping! The way they destroy the body when they are used internally, as many of them are, is that they can **(1)** suppress/really *slow down* the immune system or **(2)** actually <u>destroy</u> your internal police/immune system. For example, in the case of Lupus, a doctor may prescribe a drug that will only suppress/slow down or destroy the immune system but do NOTHING to correct the underlying problem.

Analogy 1: *Let us say that one day, all of a sudden, a normally well-behaved child starts throwing a temper tantrum and pulling dishes out of the kitchen cabinet and breaking them against the kitchen counter, knocking vases in the living room onto the floor and just messing up the entire house in general. What does the parent(s) decide to do? Pick up the kicking and screaming child, take it to its bedroom, and lock it inside. The child is still kicking and screaming in there, by the way, but at least the house is safe now...right? But what if the temper tantrum continues for days, weeks, months, years? What is the parent going to do, leave the child locked up in the room for the rest of its life? No! The parent will eventually have to let the child out, if for no other reason than to eat, because they cannot starve the child!* This is an example of <u>*suppressing or severely slowing*</u> down the immune system or covering up inflammation without trying to find the cause.

Analogy 2: In the second case of actually <u>*DESTROYING*</u> your immune system these drugs can often KILL your internal police/Immune cells in Digestion city. In fact, some steroids **kill many different types** of immune/defense cells. This is like a bomb that drops on your Army, Navy and Air Force bases as well as on the local police precincts! This can leave the United States of You open for attack by invaders! Anyone with a boat, plane or who is landlocked with the United States can just come in and take over! On the other hand, what about your crazy neighbor who wants your new car? He can just walk over and steal it now, and unless you are strong enough to stop him there is NOTHING you can do because you do not have any police/defense system now! In health, "invaders" would be bugs like viruses, bacteria and fungi! If you suppress or destroy the immune system too much you can die from the common cold!

Remembering the analogy with the child/your immune system, using a steroid would be like deciding to just lock the child away forever or to just kill the child so that you can have "peace and quiet" in your house. Again, this is not a good solution is it?

I do not want to lock away OR kill my child/immune system! What is the solution?
The best solution would be to figure out why your originally well-behaved child/immune system began to throw a tantrum. Is the child sick, sad or confused? If so, look for the underlying cause(s) to why the child is behaving like that and then get the child the help that it NEEDS. We want to get help that does not hurt the child so that the child can go back to being normal again! Likewise in naturopathic medicine we have Nature's 9 Health Laws that you have already learned about earlier, as well as natural therapies, that can help us balance either an over active or under active immune system so that we can control long lasting inflammation—all while we investigate the underlying cause(s) of the problem! **You can do this!**

Wait, you talked about inflammation just now. What does that really mean?
Inflammation is what your body is doing to repair a problem that has happened in the body. **Analogy:** *imagine you are driving down the highway and all of a sudden, (BAM!) two cars get into a car accident! We have one car on fire, two drivers hurt in their cars and all the rest of the cars on the highway have to slow down because of the accident. Whom do we need to fix this mess? We need the firefighters to put out the fires, ambulances for the hurt, police officers to direct traffic and a tow truck to take away the crashed cars. Hopefully we can get everything cleared away and running normally in as short a time as possible!*

The firefighters, police officers, ambulance and tow truck are all part of the cleanup/helping team, which is the same as what the word "inflammation" means in the body. Do you understand it? Inflammation is what your body is doing to help repair damage inside or around the body. Now, obviously if the police/firemen/tow truck/ambulance stay ALL DAY on that highway it is going to back up traffic really, really badly right? But usually they work fast and the roadway is cleared up in an hour or less depending on how much damage there is. If you have a short-term illness like a cold or flu then you will have only short-term inflammation that may last a few days or a week.

Two questions to ask with inflammation that lasts a long time in the body.
With the car accident example above, if the workers cannot clear up the damage/inflammation in a reasonable amount of time, then you have to ask yourself **(1)** why is the clean up taking so long? Are the firefighters running out of water, or does the ambulance have a flat tire? In addition **(2)** WHAT caused the accident in the first place? Was driver #1 distracted by a cell phone or maybe had their dog jumping around in the car with them, or was it that driver#2 was drunk or sleepy? Likewise with long-term inflammation in the body, we want to find out what is the underlying cause(s) of it instead of just killing or suppressing/locking away the immune system. No matter what the name of the disease, if it lasts for

weeks, months or years then you will have long-term inflammation in the United States of You. *That would be like the firemen/ambulance/police blocking two lanes of a major highway for weeks, months or years because they are unable to clear the accident! Just imagine the traffic nightmare!* ☹ Causes would then be the usual potential causes like environmental, mental/emotional, physical, or nutritional stressors and of course, ultimately that the United States of You has gotten out of tune with Nature's 9 Health Laws.

ANTACIDS

Last, but certainly not least of the three drugs I hate the most. These drugs are bad because depending on the brand, they either slow down your stomach's ability to make stomach acid or even TOTALLY STOP your stomach's ability to make stomach acid! You read earlier in Digestion chapter 4 the importance of stomach acid in killing sneaky "bugs" that try to invade the United States of You by hiding on your food and drink as you eat it. If stomach acid is lacking, that can set you up to get many infections because then these bugs can just come in as often as they like!
Analogy 1: *this is like giving the local police the night off so that criminals can take over the streets!* Also stomach acid is necessary for digestion and without Digestion city the rest of the United States of You starves!
Analogy 2: *cutting off stomach acid is like stopping the flow of gas to the engine of your car! The car CANNOT run without it!* Therefore, frequent symptoms will be bloating, indigestion and diarrhea to name a few.

In conventional medicine, often when people get heartburn it is blamed on having too much stomach acid. That is certainly a possibility, but without testing how much stomach acid you actually make, how can we know for sure? Instead of testing stomach acid, most patients get an antacid prescription for their irritating heartburn. However, did you know that you could also get heartburn because of TOO LITTLE stomach acid? YES! *I know your mouth hangs open in surprise now.*

So how does the food and stomach acid thing normally work anyway?

The way it works is that you have a sphincter/door at the bottom of your esophagus/mouth to stomach tube that sends food from your mouth to your stomach. When the food arrives, the door opens letting the food into the stomach and then the door/sphincter closes again so that neither food NOR stomach acid go back up into your throat by mistake. Stomach acid is Hydrochloric Acid/HCL a **VERY** strong chemical and it can SERIOUSLY burn you, if it gets into areas that it should not be like into your throat or into Small Intestine city! **Fact:** *Did you know that the average pH/strength of stomach acid on an empty stomach is 2-3? The LOWER the pH number the STRONGER the acid strength, so if you were to dip your finger into a jar of pH 2 stomach acid/HCL it would BURN YOUR FINGER OFF!*

But Stomach city is built to hold stomach acid and so the acid usually does not hurt the stomach, unless of course the stomach is damaged itself.

There is always a little stomach acid in your stomach, even if there is no food in there...for just in case you decide to surprise the stomach with food outside of meal times. Then when you eat, the pH/stomach acid strength increases some so that we do not burn the small intestine with acid when the food moves into there.

How does low stomach acid cause heartburn?
This is actually very common and happens because the sphincter/door does not know that it needs to stay closed because the stomach acid is not at the proper level to remind the door to stay closed. ***Analogy: have you heard of the Venus Flytrap Plant? It is a plant that has a big "mouth" that stays open all the time, UNTIL a fly or another insect flies too close to the plant's "mouth". The bug's movement is a signal to the Flytrap plant that it needs to close its mouth so suddenly whoosh! The Flytrap closes its "mouth" and eats the insect! Sorry little insect, but we all have to eat.*☹ This is how the sphincter/door works too. Normally having ENOUGH stomach acid would keep the sphincter door closed...but if there is not ENOUGH acid/insects around then the sphincter door/flytrap plant may stay open a little bit and allow stomach acid to rise up into the esophagus/mouth to stomach tube.

      In nature, an open Venus Flytrap plant is not a problem--except for the insects--but in the United States of You it is a HUGE problem because that open door can cause stomach acid to leave Stomach city and flow back up into Esophagus county and burn/set the workers on fire there! It irritates the Esophagus county workers so much, that they could decide to protest and they make so much noise that they bother the workers in nearby Lung city and this can make you cough! Especially at night when you are lying down because it is easier for stomach acid to flow back up into Esophagus county due to the law of gravity. Gravity is less with you lying down! Over years, this can even lead to cancer of the Esophagus!

Can other things beside low stomach acid affect my sphincter door and cause heartburn?
Yes, many other things can also negatively affect your sphincter/door. Examples are caffeine, eating a meal and then lying down, or even certain foods like citrus, chocolate or tomatoes. Again, the idea is to look for the cause of YOUR heartburn (it will not be the same cause for everyone) and not just to turn off stomach acid! Keep the "gas" flowing to your "engine"!

DRUGS THAT STEAL VITAMINS AND MINERALS

Many prescribed or over the counter medications can leach or pull vitamins and minerals out of your body! The same way that a leech sucks your blood out. ☹

Here is just a tiny list. It does not include all drugs or all vitamins/minerals that are leached out nor all the medical issues that can be caused. That would make this book MUCH longer. ☹ For a more complete list, see the Drug Induced Nutrient Depletion Handbook.[55]

Drug Type	Nutrient Deficiency	Potential Health Issue
Antacids or **Anti-ulcer**	Vitamin B12	anemia/tired and weak, hand tremors
	Folic Acid	birth defects, problems in all organs/cities
	Vitamin D	weak: bones, muscles and teeth
	Calcium	weak bones and teeth, heart problems
	Iron	anemia/tired and weak
	Zinc	low immune system
Antibiotics	B Vitamins	MANY ISSUES! Low energy
	Vitamin K	weak bones; tendency to bleeding
	Calcium	dementia and depression
	Magnesium	heart problems, Premenstrual Syndrome
	Iron	shortness of breath
	Vitamin B6	low energy, poor mental function
	Zinc	poor wound healing
Cholesterol Lowering Drugs	Coenzyme Q10	heart problems
Antidepressants	Coenzyme Q10	low energy
Female Hormones	B Vitamins	depression, sleeping problems
	Vitamin C	frequent cold/flu and easy bruising
	Magnesium	bone problems, muscle cramps
	Selenium	low immune system
Anticonvulsants (anti-seizure)	Vitamin D and Calcium	weak immune system; cataracts
	Folic Acid and Biotin	low energy; bad skin and hair loss
	Selenium and Zinc	thyroid problems; slow growth (kids)
	Carnitine	heart problems, low energy

Drug Type	Nutrient Deficiency	Potential Health Issue
Anti-inflammatories	Calcium and Vitamin D	weak muscles; blood pressure problems
	Magnesium and Zinc	asthma; skin problems
	Vitamins B6 and B12	depression; muscle twitches/shakes
	Selenium and Iron	poor ability to detox; weak hair and nails
	Chromium	high: blood sugar, cholesterol, triglycerides
	Vitamins C and B5	slow wound healing; low energy
Diuretics (water removing pills)	Potassium	irregular heartbeat, fatigue, weak muscles
	Vitamins B1 and B6	low energy; memory loss, sleep problems
	Calcium and Zinc	muscle cramps; bad or slow sperm
	Sodium	dehydration, muscle weakness
	Magnesium	heart and muscle problems
	Folic Acid	birth defects and many other things
Heart medications Blood pressure etc.	Coenzyme Q10	brain and nerve problems
	Vitamins B1 and B6	depression; irritability
	Zinc	weak or poor sense of smell and taste
Diabetes Drugs	Coenzyme Q10	yes... again. ☹
	Vitamin B12	heart problems, nerve problems
Anti-viral Drugs	Calcium and Zinc	tooth decay; low testosterone
	Copper	joint problems and low energy
	Carnitine	abnormal blood sugar and liver function

Wow. That was depressing.☹ Remember that **EACH** of the nutrients that I listed here does *AT LEAST* 4 different things in the body! Some of them like Vitamin D and Zinc do over 20 things! These medications are stealing nutrients (vitamins and minerals) that you need! *Analogy: that is like you working hard and putting $20 in your wallet and every time you put money in the wallet a thief comes along and steals the $20 out of it!*

Again, you may need to take one or two of these medications at one time or another for a brief period. However, you can see that taking them also weakens many other areas in the body. You can refer back to the Nature's 9 Health Laws chapter under the nutrition section to see what certain vitamins and minerals do in the body. When these vitamins/minerals are lacking or these medications pull them out of the body, your health will only get worse! That is why you should be trying to get back in tune with Nature's 9 Health Laws so that you can be healthy completely!

CHAPTER 14: So besides drugs and surgery what natural therapies can I use?

There are numerous natural therapies that can help the body to heal itself. In naturopathic medical school we study and train extensively in the top seven. Each one of these therapies has at least five or six classes behind it!

SEVEN MAIN NATURAL THERAPIES

(1) **Acupuncture/Acupressure & Traditional Chinese Medicine Diagnosis and techniques**
(2) Botanical/Herbal Medicine
(3) **Clinical Nutrition and Food Sensitivities**
(4) Environmental Medicine
(5) **Homeopathic Medicines**
(6) Mind & Body Medicine
(7) **Physical Medicine**

All of the following natural therapies can be used to stimulate a certain area/part/organ and help the ENTIRE body to rebuild and restore health to itself. Therefore, you can use these natural therapies for short-term illness--colds, flus, aches, pains and long-term illness such as Diabetes, Heart disease, and Cancer. Although you can use them alone, in general, the more natural therapies that are combined in a targeted and systematic way, the more powerful the healing!

NATUROPATHIC MEDICINE: 7 MAIN THERAPIES

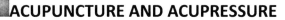

ACUPUNCTURE AND ACUPRESSURE

Acupuncture: uses tiny, strategically placed needles along certain points on the body to help stimulate parts/organs to regain function. Do not worry, typically you do not feel the needles at all and usually there is no blood either! There is no scarring or tattooing with this procedure. **Acupressure:** uses the same points but no needles. *Using needles is more effective though, so do not be scared!*

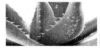 **BOTANICAL/HERBAL MEDICINE**

(my second favorite therapy☺)

Using plants/plant parts to rebuild the body. Plants can be used:
(1) orally in teas, supplements or tinctures/high concentration liquid form
(2) applied onto the body using water/oil/lotion/cream based applications
(3) inhaled using essential oils or steam inhalation treatments. One type of lesser-known botanical medicine is the use of flower essences. A great company is Lotus Wei flower essences.[44]

 CLINICAL NUTRITION/FOOD SENSITIVITIES

Obviously eating a bad/unhealthy diet will destroy your health—and MANY of us are sick because we eat poorly, but even some good foods can make you feel badly! Your body may HATE oranges and that could be making you sick—*but seriously, it is probably all of the junk or the sheer amount of food you eat that is making you sick and not the oranges.* We cannot all eat the same diet! This area teaches you what to eat, when to eat it, how much to eat, and how often. Learn what nutrition plan is right for YOU.

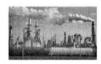 **ENVIRONMENTAL MEDICINE**

Pesticides on food. Drugs in our drinking water. Air pollution. Our bodies are always under attack! This teaches where toxins come from and how to help your body kick them OUT!

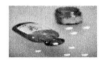 **HOMEOPATHIC MEDICINE**

These medicines work a lot like vaccines do: use a little bit of a substance to prepare your body to fight (and win) against a bigger problem!

 MIND BODY MEDICINE & COUNSELING

Uses therapists to help train the mind to uncover or recognize a scary or hurtful memory/event and then strives to change how the mind and body react to that memory/event.

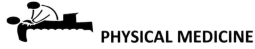 **PHYSICAL MEDICINE**

Structure affects function! Just like driving a car with only three wheels is going to make your car scrape, drag and clunk down the road, having your spine, bones and muscles out of alignment can make your other organs not work properly! This therapy physically moves parts around for perfect function. Brain city is really involved with this therapy so it is great!

Let us not stop now! More natural healing therapies exist!
19 MORE TYPES OF NATURAL THERAPIES!
I am so excited therefore I will type this phrase AGAIN and even bigger! ☺

19 MORE TYPES OF NATURAL THERAPIES!

This list is certainly not all-inclusive but reflects the majority of natural therapies that are possible. Many of these therapies such as physical medicine, hydrotherapy, massage, physiotherapy machines, and Chinese medicine techniques have MULTIPLE different type therapies under their name so actually there are more than 40 natural therapies listed! Additionally, the uses noted are just a few of the most common uses but many more are possible!
Do you know about these?

ANIMAL THERAPY 1
Uses: mental/emotional traumas, post-traumatic stress disorder, depression
Why it works: trained animals can BOTH stimulate and calm the brain in ways humans cannot!

AROMA THERAPY 2
Uses: lung infections, anxiety, panic, depression
Why it works: plants with volatile oils travel directly back to the brain and lungs to effect healing!

CRANIO SACRAL THERAPY 3
Uses: migraines, neck/back pain, Autism, traumatic brain and spinal cord injuries, after surgery *and more!*
Why it works: using a super light touch enhances the body's healing power

CHIROPRACTIC/PHYSICAL MEDICINE 4
Uses: neck/back pain, hearing loss, digestive complaints, after physical trauma, balance problems
Why it works: by relaxing tight muscles & realigning the spine, the organs work as they should
Different types: Trigger point therapy/neuromuscular technique (NMT) range of motion, compression and traction exercises, muscle energy technique, applied kinesiology

CRYOTHERAPY 5
Uses: body wide inflammation, skin lesions, muscle soreness and certain cancers
Why it works: exposing a part or the entire body to below zero temperatures for a few minutes propels the body to decrease harmful factors and promotes healing.

HYDROTHERAPY 6 *my favorite therapy of all!* ☺
Uses: EVERYTHING! Digestive complaints, cancer, high blood pressure, cold/flu
Why it works: we use water for healing! Hot water brings blood to an area of the body, cold drives blood away. However, depending on how hot or cold the temperature of the water, and how long we apply the water, we can direct blood flow to places all around the body. *That is like being able to control the traffic lights and yield/stop signs as you are driving!*
Different types: alternating hot and cold in the shower; constitutional, whirlpool, neutral baths, fever baths, warming sheet wrap, enemas, Russian steam wrap, sauna, warming socks, topical applications to body parts or steam inhalation using herbs...*seriously, I could go on and on and on here...some one stop me!*

INFRARED SAUNA 7
Uses: high blood pressure, pain relief, detoxification, and to improve blood circulation
Why it works: the body responds to heat which speed up the body's ability to get rid of harmful toxins!

LIGHT THERAPY 8
Uses: detoxification, relaxation, organ damage restoration
Why it works: certain wavelengths of full spectrum light shining through theatrical gels, or from specially formulated lightbulbs can stimulate the body to perform certain functions such as lemon or dark green light for detoxifying, or pale violet light for healing!

MASSAGE 9
Uses: muscle/neck/back pain, help inner organs cleanse toxins, constipation
Why it works: light or deep touch stimulates the area to enhance its function.
Types: Lymphatic, Deep Organ, Swedish, Reflexology

MAGNETIC THERAPY[22] 10
Uses: pain, nerve and muscle damage, decreased energy and much more!
Why it works: the body has magnetic fields that can become unbalanced and placing magnets in specific areas can realign the unbalanced magnetic poles!
Types: Shoe insoles, necklaces, bracelets, blankets, sitting pads

MIND BODY MEDICINE TECHNIQUES 11
Uses: post-traumatic stress disorders, anxiety, panic attacks, phobias
Why it works: it uses techniques or a machine to show how your body is negatively reacting to a negative thought or memory—such as your heart rate or a harmful brain wave is increasing. Then the therapist coaches you to change the thought and reaction from a negative to a positive or less harmful reaction. You can see your improvement in real time with Biofeedback and Neurofeedback!
Types: Meditation, Neurofeedback, Biofeedback, Eye Movement Desensitization and Reprocessing/EMDR.

MUSIC THERAPY 12
Uses: post-traumatic stress disorder, memory loss, dementia/Alzheimer's
Why it works: music is a powerful tool in the brain; it can arouse emotion as well as relax the senses. Even those with Alzheimer's can recall childhood songs!

Nambudripad's Allergy Elimination Technique/NAET[18] 13
Uses: ALLERGIES! Environmental (animal dander, trees etc.), food and chemical allergy sources
Why it works: using nutrients, physical manipulations and other natural, non-invasive treatments over a series of sessions, one can retrain the body to overcome allergies.

PHYSIOTHERAPY MACHINES[19] **14**
Uses: pain (muscle or nerve), paralysis, speed wound healing--broken bones/strains/sprains, arthritis, skin infections, enhance blood/lymph flow, increase protein production in body, decrease scarring after surgery, sluggish organs.
Why it works: these machines operate in different ways: some use heat or cold, light waves, sound waves, electrical or magnetic fields, sine wave or minerals/ions. Some act on a cellular/deep level or some in a more broad/superficial sense but in general, each will stimulate the area of the body to which they are applied by helping bring nutrients to the area and helping the body remove trash/toxins from an area!
Different types: Diathermy, Sine Wave, High or Low Voltage Galvanism, Iontophoresis, Cold Laser, Interferential, Microcurrent, TENS/Transcutaneous Electrical Nerve Stimulation, Infrared Light Lamp, Ultraviolet light, Phonophoresis and Ultrasound-*it is not just for looking at unborn babies* ☺

PROLOTHERAPY 15 (nonsurgical tendon/ligament reconstruction) [20]
Uses: facial muscle/jaw pain, arthritis, joint pain, back pain, sports injuries of the muscles or joints.
Why it works: with prolotherapy using repetitive injections of non-harmful substances--often from the individual's own body, such as platelets, or dextrose/a natural sugar or certain minerals—can stimulate the body to regenerate/heal naturally! *Much healthier than using steroid injections!*
Types: Dextrose, Platelet Rich Plasma, Bio Cellular prolotherapy.

SENSORY DEPRIVATION THERAPY/FLOTATION TANKS/Restricted Environmental Stimulation Technique (R.E.S.T) [21] **16**
Uses: high blood pressure, pain, muscle/nerve healing, relaxation...EVERYTHING!
Why it works: being inside a lightless, soundproof tank floating in high salinity/salt water at skin temperature allows the brain to almost completely relax and not have to work so hard processing all of the typical stimulants of sound, touch, temperature and light thereby leading to healing!

TOPICAL APPLICATIONS/PROCEDURES 17
Uses: arthritis, joint pain/stiffness, poor circulation/cold hands and feet, facial muscle problems, organ cleansing and healing (castor oil cloth)
Why it works: using wax, heat or cold can increase blood flow to areas to remove trash/toxins and bring in needed nutrients like vitamins and minerals!
Types: Paraffin Bath/wax, Cold Friction Spray/Vapo-coolant, Skin Brushing, Castor Oil Cloth

TRADITIONAL CHINESE MEDICINE TECHNIQUES 18 *(my third favorite!☺)*
Uses: EVERYTHING! Pain ANYWHERE; any slow/badly functioning organ/city or part of body.
Why it works: in order below, these use: heat, slowly and fluidly moving your body posture/breathing, scraping the body, electric current, heated herbs placed on body, massage/body work, and needles placed in strategic places to stimulate muscles, nerves and organs to regenerate and perform their functions!
Different types: Cupping, Qi Gong, Gua Sha, Electrotherapy, Moxibustion, Tui Na, and of course Acupuncture (uses needles) and Acupressure (without needles)...*not to mention many more!*

OXYGEN THERAPIES 19[45]
Uses: ANY DISEASE! SHORT-TERM or LONG-TERM.
Why it works: we need oxygen as an energy source for basic function and for healing of any organ/city or part of the body.
Different types: (1) with Hyperbaric Oxygen Therapy/HBOT you lie inside a pressurized and oxygenated enclosed area that looks like a big clear capsule for two hours. This is done in a physician's office or clinic and requires multiple sessions. **(2)** With Live O2 oxygen therapy, you wear an oxygen mask and breathe deeply while you are pedaling on a stationary bike for minimum 15 minutes. This is done in a doctor's office or clinic or you can purchase the equipment and do the treatments at home.

WOW! I HAD NO IDEA SO MANY NON-DRUG/NON SURGERY NATURAL THERAPIES EXISTED!

Those were my same thoughts as I was studying about these while in naturopathic medical school! It is amazing! There are even more! So consider *NOT* covering up or living with symptoms. Consider *NOT* cutting out some part of your body, and leaving an empty space there; or replacing it with something worse or not as good as what you were born with. **Example:** like getting a metal knee versus healing YOUR knee or replacing your heart or kidney with someone else's! Think about (and DO) these options first while you are also getting back in tune with Nature's 9! **You can do this!**

CHAPTER 15: My ten favorite home therapies for colds, flu and more!

Many of you catch colds/flus and stomach bugs and you do not have a clue of how you can use some of the natural medicines and home therapies to help your body restore health to itself so I wanted to include a few of my favorite therapies. Here they are in no particular order... I love and use them ALL.☺

Number 1: STEAM INHALATION TREATMENT
What you can use it for: colds/flus, sinus headaches, nasal congestion, dry cough or cough with phlegm/mucus, sinus problems, just cleaning out your lungs after exposure to chemical fumes like cigarette smoke, new paint/new carpet off gassing or even if you have a job where you are exposed to fumes.

Why it works: These herbs are antimicrobial/fight bugs (viruses, bacteria, fungi) and have volatile oils in them that are activated by the high heat, so that when you breathe them in, the oils travel through your nose and into Lung city and kill the evil bugs! These herbs also just have a nice cleaning out effect in the nose and lungs even if you are not sick. Eucalyptus is an herb with an affinity to the lung, meaning Eucalyptus LOVES to travel to the lung versus anywhere else in the body!

How to do it: You need Thyme, Rosemary and Eucalyptus. Or at least 2 of any combination of the three herbs: so Thyme and Eucalyptus or Rosemary and Eucalyptus. One herb alone can work ok, but it is best to have at least two. Buy bulk herbs--loose herbs in jars, not tea bags—of course if you cannot find bulk herbs use what you can find. Change herbs after two uses. Bring a covered pot of 4 cups of water and 4 tablespoons of each herb to boiling. *Keep the lid on the pot at all times. We are trying to catch steam!* At boil turn off fire. Place the pot onto a food tray or place the pot on your lap. You can also do the treatment by standing and leaning over the stove. *Entire family sick? Make a "tent" in the living room!* ☺

Get a large towel or sheet and cover your head and the covered pot completely. Wrap the sheet under your arms and around the tray/drape it down your legs. *We do not want steam to escape!* Now uncover the lid, lean slightly over into the pot (careful not to burn your face) and breathe in the steam from the pot by deeply breathing through your nose. If your nose is congested, you can breathe in through your mouth too. You can take short breaks if you become overheated. Cover the pot while you are on break. Try to stay under the sheet/towel as long as possible. Try to breathe the steam for 5 minutes minimum. If you are claustrophobic and do not want to cover your head and body you do not have to do so. Just place your face as close to the pot as possible.

How often to do it: can do it once, twice or multiple times a day until the symptoms go away and then one day past that. Remember, you can also do it as needed, like if you had to spend the day near someone who smokes and you want to clean out your lungs and nose a little.

Number 2: ALTERNATING HYDROTHERAPY IN THE SHOWER. *My favorite!* ☺
What you can use it for: high blood pressure, back/neck/chest pain, cold hands/feet, EVERYTHING!
Why it works: *increases movement of blood circulation/semi-trucks. Heat brings blood to the surface of an area, cold takes blood away from the area initially, but then cold sends it back to nourish the area for longer than heat so the COLD is the best part to restore health--do not skip it!*

How to do it: 4 cycles minimum but you can do as many as you like! While in the shower stand with your chest in water stream. Use hot water as hot as you can stand it without burning skin for 2 minutes, then switch to cold water—all the way cold if you can--for 30 seconds. Repeat on your back. That is one cycle. Repeat cycles as above. Should take about 10 minutes. *You need to be VERY warm/hot from doing the hot water part BEFORE beginning the cold water part, meaning do not move onto the cold part if you really are not warm after the first hot part. So continue the first hot part for longer than 2 minutes or until you are really warm/hot then proceed to first cold portion and subsequent cycles. We NEVER add more cold to an already cold person!* ☹ *However, keep in mind that the reason this works is that there is a temperature difference, so we want VERY hot water versus VERY cold water. If your shower does not become hot enough or cold enough then you may want to try alternating hot and cold therapy using two different pots and two different wash cloths. The two pots method also works well if you are working on a specific area like a hurt knee or something.*

How often to do it: can do it daily, twice a day or a few days a week, the more the better! But do not run up your water bill, once a day while you are showering is enough, unless you are very ill and then twice a day is best. ☺

Number 3: CASTOR OIL CLOTH *You can purchase castor oil from health food stores/pharmacies. The Heritage Store brand is a good one. Cold pressed. Castor oil is <u>SUPER POWERFUL! IT IS NOT JUST AN OILY RAG</u>!* **My 3rd favorite!** ☺
What you can use it for: constipation; upset stomach for when you ate too much or ate something that does not agree with you; joint pain, back pain and MORE!

Why it works: Castor oil over the abdomen/stomach increases semi-trucks/blood circulation to Stomach city. It increases trash removal via bowel movements in Large Intestine/Colon city! It also helps with pain in many areas so you can use it on fingers/wrists/knees/ankles or on the back for pain in those areas too!

How to do it: Soak a washcloth in castor oil until fully wet and practically dripping. Cover stomach*. Leave over stomach for 30 minutes minimum. However, you can even sleep with it overnight! Watch for discomfort the first time using it over the stomach or low abdomen. *Optional: you can use wax paper to cover the castor oil cloth and then add a heating pad over wax paper to increase how much goes into your skin.* Do not let castor oil touch your clothes/sheets or furniture because it will leave an oil stain! If you decide to sleep with it on your back, protect your bed sheets by first laying down an old towel/sheet or shirt, then laying down wax paper or parchment paper and then place the soaked cloth on top of that. *If using castor oil on a hand or ankle/leg then soak a glove/sock or small strip of cloth in castor oil and then wear the glove/sock/strip around the hurting joint for the same amount of time or even longer! After you finish just place the cloth in a little bowl.

How often to do it: minimum four consecutive days, less than that and we do not really see an effect. You do not wash the cloth! You just keep on adding oil to it before each use so that it is soaked. The idea is that the cloth must always be almost dripping before every use. The cloth will last for months or a year!

Number 4: SKIN BRUSHING *You can get a skin brush from a health food store or use a damp washcloth*
What you can use it for: colds, flus, and any long term illness, or even just to stay healthy!
Why it works: this helps to move lymph fluid/trucks on side roads around
How to do it: always brush in the direction of the heart--which is in the top left corner of your chest. Brush over your stomach--brush upwards--minimum 30 strokes. Brush under your jaw, each side of your neck and under arms 10 strokes each side (brush downwards). Brush on the inside of both legs (brush upwards)
How often to do it: daily would be great, or three times a week.

Number 5: FEVER BATH
What you can use it for: cold or flu
Why it works: using heating herbs creates a "fake" fever which makes the police/immune system cells drive faster to the problem area. **Analogy:** *like the difference between when you see police driving down the road at a normal speed versus when they FLY past you at 90 miles an hour with sirens and blue lights!*

How to do it
(1) Get three herbs: mustard powder, ginger powder, cayenne powder.
(2) Put two tablespoons of each herb into a thin sock and tie a knot/use string around the head of a sock to keep the herbs inside. Fill the bathtub with hot water as hot as you can stand it...VERY HOT! However, do not burn yourself. Use petroleum jelly or some kind of oil around knees, private parts and nipples to protect them.
(3) Put the herb sock into the water and squeeze the sock for two to three minutes so that the herbs begin to diffuse into water. The water color should change.
(4) Get into the tub and drink five cups of WARM WATER with lemon OR warm water with 1 tablespoon of ginger powder.
(5) Soak in the tub for minimum 20 minutes and drink ALL of the fluid while in the tub.
(6) After 20 minutes, empty the water, stand up SLOWLY and turn on the cold water from the shower. Rinse with COLD water only for 1 minute.
(7) Dry off quickly.
How often to do it: once or twice a week until you are better.

Number 6: WARMING SOCKS
What you can use it for: chest congestion with cold or flu
Why it works: having "cold feet" attracts blood there so that the blood can warm the feet up. As the blood is leaving the lungs on its way south to the feet, it "drags" mucus and trash out of the lungs!
How to do it: get a pair of cotton socks. Soak the socks in cold water and then completely ring out ALL of the water. Place the wet socks in the freezer for at least two hours. At bedtime, remove the socks from the freezer and put them on your feet. Then put one pair of dry WOOL socks over the frozen socks--or two pairs of DRY cotton socks if you cannot find wool socks. Wool is better because it handles moisture better than cotton. Wrap up the rest of your body VERY well! Wear warm pajamas and then put extra layers on top of that like wear sweat pants and a sweat shirt(s) over the pajamas and then maybe a bathrobe. The point is *you need to have AT LEAST 2-3 LAYERS of warm clothing on since you have freezing socks on your feet or else **you will make yourself sicker!*** Cover yourself with a blanket. Go to sleep. *(Sweet dreams...zzzzzzzz).*Your body should warm the cold wet socks to completely dry within 2-4 hours. If you wake up in the middle of the night and the socks are dry then your body has done its job and you can remove the socks and some of your extra layers. If you wake up in the night and the socks are STILL wet, your body is not working as well as it should be! Remove the wet socks, put on dry ones and go back to sleep and do some of the other cold and flu suggestions.
How often to do it: nightly until better

Number 7: AIR BATH

What you can use it for: get toxins/trash out of your body: allergies, skin infections.

Why it works: Skin city is the largest organ that is *outside* of the United States of You and is constantly being "smothered" in clothing...clothing that often is toxic because of dyes and chemicals in the clothes! So let it breathe!

How to do it: following shower, dry off. If you are more conservative, stay in the bathroom and then sit completely naked, for at least 5-15 min. You can read a book or magazine if you like. If non-conservative then you can walk around the house or your bedroom! If you can get some exposure to fresh air and sunlight on your skin from a window then that would be even better! Just do not give a naked peep show to the neighbors. ☹

How often to do it: daily would be great for 5 minutes, but even twice a week for 20 minutes or once a week for 30 minutes would be helpful!

Number 8: ACTIVATED CHARCOAL *(not charcoal from the grill!)*

What you can use it for: insect bites, bee stings, spider bites; pulling toxins out of Digestion city.

Why it works: it draws out bad "bug juice" from under your skin that those mean insects put in there. That is what makes your skin swell and itch and turn red! It also helps pull toxins out of Digestion city by "grabbing" them and when you poop the toxins are stuck to the charcoal!

How to do it: open up 2-3 capsules. Mix with a little water to form a paste then apply it to the bug bite and cover with a bandage. Leave it on for a few hours. *Do not put it over cut skin*! If using it for Digestion city, you can put about 1 teaspoon in eight ounces or 1 cup/250 mL of water and drink.

Where to get it: from a local health food store or online store like Vitacost.

Number 9: BENTONNITE CLAY

What you can use it for: arthritis; nerve illnesses like Multiple Sclerosis *and more!*

Why it works: It pulls toxins out of the body through Skin city

How to do it: in a bowl, mix a few tablespoons of clay with enough water to make a thin paste. Get an old sheet. Lay down on the sheet and spread the paste all over the main area you are working on: legs, arms, stomach, back or you can do the whole body. Lay on sheet for at least an hour. *Watch TV, nap or read a book.* ☺ Then wash off the clay completely in the shower. Do this at least once or twice a week. Can do it daily.

Where to get it: from a local health food store or online store like Vitacost.

Number 10: ENEMA
What you can use it for: colds, flus, a day or two with no bowel movement
Why it works: the water stimulates or "pokes" the large intestine muscles so that you can have a bowel movement/BM/poop. When you are sick with a cold or flu, you make even more "trash" so you want to help your body get rid of it. On the other hand, if you have not pooped in a few days you do not want to keep building up trash so this helps the body throw it away.

How to do it: Lay a towel on the bathroom floor. Fill the enema bag with 2-4 cups of water only. Lie on your left side. Insert the tube 2-3 inches into the rectum. Be sure to put some oil or petroleum jelly around the end of the tube so that it slides in smoothly. Let the water start flowing in. Hold the bag up as high as you can with your arm so that water flows faster. Once all the water is inside you, remove the tube and lay the enema bag down. Stay on the floor for 3-5 minutes and massage your belly/abdomen in a clockwise direction. Afterwards, get on the toilet and "fire away"! ☺ You may want to sit on the toilet a few extra minutes after the first poop to make sure there is nothing left over in there.

Where to get an enema bag: From a local health food store, online health food store like Vitacost or even a medical supplies store.

Note: Colon hydrotherapy is a more in depth "enema" using water and a machine. It is done in a colon hydrotherapy/wellness center or in a doctor's office. Once or twice a month you can do this if you would like. But not more often than that.

WARNING: You should not need to do enemas more than once or twice a month. If you do enemas too often the body can get "lazy" and decide not to poop on its own without the enema to stimulate/poke it. If you find that you need to use enemas more often than once or twice a month you need to look for the reason Large Intestine city is so slow. It could be because of a change in: foods, routine, exercise or something else. Then once you identify the problem, correct that problem so that you can poop normally again!

Thanks to C. Rentz for reminding me to add this therapy!

MUST HAVE HERBS AND STUFF FOR THE HOUSE!

People often ask me about which herbs (and other products) they should have in stock at all times in the house for different problems so here is my favorites list!

Herbs have a Latin name and a common name. Most people just use the **common names** but sometimes based on what region you live in the herb may have a different common name from another region in the same country or the common name may differ in a foreign country. Therefore, we use the **Latin names** so that wherever you go, you know that you have the right herb. The first name I list for the herb is the common name and the name in parentheses () will be the Latin name.

You can purchase these herbs as a highly concentrated premade liquid called a **tincture** or you can buy **bulk** herbs. That means that the herb is in a big jar--not in a tea bag--and you tell them how many ounces you want to buy. Keep in mind that most tinctures are made with alcohol. There is only a *tiny* amount of alcohol left in there and tinctures are perfectly safe for most people. With many plants, we must use alcohol to get to the helpful parts because the elements we need will not come out of the plant using only water. **RESOURCE:** buy herbs online at Mountain Rose Herbs[77].

However, if the person who will use the tincture is a recovering alcoholic or a child then you can look for that same tincture but instead use one made from a **glycerite** meaning they did not use alcohol to make it. A glycerite tincture is labeled as such on the front of the bottle.

You do not have to buy all the herbs I have listed but try to have at least **two herbs** from each category; herbs work well alone but work better if there are two or more.

Analogy: *it is ok to have just a mom or just a dad but to have TWO parents is best!*

Depending on where you shop, you may be able to find some herbs better than others. My **favorite** two herbs under each section will have a star*.

Plant parts: We can use different parts of the plant for different things, and sometimes a certain plant part is stronger or better than another part of the plant. For example, the berry from a plant might be better for lowering blood pressure than the leaf from that same plant. Some stores carry only one plant part at a time and then change parts. Therefore, when you are looking to buy an herb/plant one day you might find the root and another day only the powder. The best general rule is that plant roots and leaves are always better than the powder form of that plant.

Once we turn a plant into a powder, it can more easily start rotting (oxidizing) than if you leave it intact. So avoid using powders. But if there is nothing else then just buy that. **Avoid buying herbs in tea bags**. The herbs could be very old or have dead insects in the bags and you would not even know.☹

Tea preparation: Put 1-3 tablespoons of each herb into about 4 (eight ounce) cups/1 liter of water and bring to a boil. Once at a boil, turn off the heat and let the herbs steep/stay in the water for at least one hour before using. Most of the herbs from the list below you use as a tea. The skin herbs are mainly to be used directly on the skin topically/on the outside/not drunk in a tea.

Note: Most items on this list are herbs, however if it is a supplement or other product, I listed the brand name that I prefer first, and then the product name. For example, Zyflamend is a product that one can use for aching, stiff joints. New Chapter is the brand or company that makes it and Zyflamend is the name of the product. You can buy most of the *products* either locally or on an online health food store such as Vitacost or even on Amazon. Sometimes the companies make you order the products through your doctor. The herbs you can find in a local health food store.

Last thing: these symbols ! ^ # ^^ in front of an herb or item mean that there are more notes about the herb/product at the end. ☺

STRESS
Rhodiola root (Rhodiola rosacea)*
Ashwaganda (Withania somnifera)*
Holy Basil (Ocimum sanctum)
Schisandra berry (Schisandra chinensis)
Coleus root (Coleus forskholli)
Bladderwrack fronds (Fucus vesiculosis)

SLEEP
Skullcap (Scutellaria lateriflora)*
Kava Kava root (Piper Methysticum)
Passionflower (Passiflora incarnata)*
Hops (Humulus lupulus)
Chamomile (Matricaria recutita)

HEART
!Cayenne pepper (Capsicum annum)*
Hawthorn berry (Crataegus oxycantha)
Maidenhair tree (Gingko biloba)
Ginger root (Zingiber officinalis)*
Horse Chestnut (Aesculus hippocastanum)
Witch Hazel (Hamamelis virginiana)
^ Fresh garlic and onions!

LUNGS (and sinuses)
Eucalyptus (E. globulus)*
Elecampagne (Inula helenium)
Yerba Santa (Eriodictyon californicum)
Indian Tobacco (Lobelia inflata)
(Lobelia is not tobacco!)
Thyme (Thymus Vulgaris)*

DIGESTION AND LIVER
Yellow Gentian (Gentiana lutea)*
Peppermint (Mentha piperita)
Ginger (Zingiber officinalis)
Artichoke (Cynara scolymus)
Milk Thistle (Silybum marianum)*

KIDNEYS AND BLADDER
Dandelion (Taraxacum officinalis)*
Celery seed (Apium graveolens)
Parsley root (Petroselinum crispum)
Cornsilk (Zea Mays)*

SORE MUSCLES OR BRUISES
MediNatura brand T-Relief gel* or tablets
OR
Arnica Cream
Castor oil cloth (see chapter 15 number 3)*

SKIN (small cuts and scars)+++
Eastern coltsfoot (Tussilago farfara)
Vitamin E (buy oil or open capsules)*
Aloe Vera gel*
Comfrey (Symphytum officinale)

MUSCLES: CRAMPS AND OR PAIN
Hylands Brand homeopathic tablets: #8 Mag. Phos. 6X

IMMUNE SYSTEM (Colds/Flus)
Thyme (Thymus vulgaris)*
Rosemary (Rosmarinus officinalis)*
Purple Cone Flower (Echinacea)
Huang Qi (Astragalus)
^^Fresh garlic

WOUND HEALING HERBS###
Yarrow (Achillea millefolium)*
Calendula (Calendula officinalis)*
Plantain (Plantago major)
Chamomile (Matricaria recutita)

BRAIN HEALTH
Maiden hair tree (Gingko biloba)*
Gotu Kola (Centella asiatica)

ENERGY
Asian Ginseng (Panax ginseng)* *
Ginger (Zingiber officinalis)

***ANY ginseng is fine! Panax quinquefolium (American) or Eleutherococcus (Siberian).*

SEASONAL ALLERGIES   (these are all supplements)
BHI brand Allergy Relief Homeopathic dissolving tablets* *(my favorite!)*
Orthomolecular brand Natural-D-Hist*
Spring Board brand D-Hist-Jr
Protocol for Life Balance brand Aller All

JOINTS: ACHY/STIFF/PAINFUL
Tumeric (Curcuma longa)
Cayenne (Capsicum)
Castor oil cloth/sock/glove*
Supplement: Herbalist and Alchemist brand 7 Precious Mushrooms* (liquid 2 ounce)
Product: New Chapter brand Zyflamend. You can take this internally or you can actually pierce the capsule with a needle or safety pin and then squeeze out the herbal "goodness" onto your finger and rub it into the joint that hurts! Be careful though because it contains Tumeric, which can stain your clothing yellow orange! ☹.

It works fast! I actually used it myself once when I had some achy joints. I broke it open an rubbed in on my hip. It contains anti-pain herbs like Rosemary, Tumeric and Ginger. It helps decrease inflammation and promotes healing with other herbs such as Holy Basil (Ocimum sanctum), organic Green Tea (Camellia sinensis),
Hu Zhang (Polygonum cuspidatum), Chinese Goldthread (Coptis chinensis), Barberry (Berberis vulgaris), Oregano (Origanum vulgare) and Skullcap (Scutellaria baicalensis). Pronouncing some of those herbs makes your tongue twist around in your mouth! ☺

Note: if you cannot find or afford the Zyflamend product then you can get the Turmeric and Cayenne in powder form and heat up a tablespoon of each into 2 tablespoons of Olive oil. Bring to a boil. Then rub the cool mix into the joints! Cayenne will make it burn very hot! It is not damaging your skin though so do not worry. It will eventually cool down.

HAIR FORMULA
Tea Tree (Melaleuca alternifolia) use essential oil drops—*or dried herb if can't find drops*
Horse Chestnut (Aesculus hippocastanum) dried herb—*hard to find essential oil drops*
Rosemary (Rosmarinus officinalis) essential oil drops *or dried herb*
Melatonin supplement
Biotin shampoo and conditioner--*or any healthy brand shampoo/conditioner*

Heat 2 tablespoons of both Horse chestnut and Rosemary in 4 ounces/125 mL of water. Bring to boil. Turn off heat and strain herbs. To the shampoo and the conditioner add each of the following: 2 ounces/62 mL of the herb mix; open up and pour in 3 caps of Melatonin; 5-15 drops of Tea Tree (and or Rosemary) essential oils. Shake both the shampoo and conditioner well. The Tea Tree will make your head tingle but that is ok! Helps stimulate/increase hair growth!

EYE HEALTH
Bilberry (Vaccinum myrtillus) and berries in general like blueberry/strawberry
Eyebright (Euphrasia officinalis)
Zinc (not an herb, a mineral)
Lycopene (not an herb, get it from *cooked* tomatoes/tomato pastes)
Vitamin A
Carrots

Thanks to Ben O. for requesting the eye health section!

Notes
!For Cayenne pepper I do not like the powder sold in most grocery/health food stores because it is not strong enough. I recommend Dr. Richard Shulze[4] liquid or powder Cayenne. For all other herbs buying them in a health food store is ok.

^Garlic and onions are not "dried herbs" but they are super powerful for helping the heart pump better and making your blood not stick together! Using them fresh is more powerful than after you cook them.

^^Garlic again! It is fantastic at killing all bad "bugs" like viruses, bacteria, and fungi! One of my favorite "I am sick recipes" is a Garlic drink.

- 4 ounces/125 mL of Orange juice or Apple juice (no added sugar)
- 4 ounces/125 mL of water
- 1 Tablespoon/14 mL of Olive oil
- 3 cloves of fresh Garlic

Blend everything in a blender OR if you are very brave, just chop the Garlic very small (or put through a garlic press) and then throw it into a cup with the liquid ingredients and then drink/chew and swallow!

+++Skin healing herbs use these ON the skin. Do not use internally/swallow them. They will not kill you; it is just that we want them to go directly on the skin without having to go all through your digestive system and body first!

###Wound healing herbs help your body heal from inside wounds--like after physical trauma or surgery--as well as wounds on the outside like cuts and bruises. For internal wounds, you can make a tea and drink it and for external wounds, you can drink some of the tea AND soak a thin clean rag in the rest of the tea, wring out the cloth—remove all herb pieces*--and then place the cloth onto the wound! **DO NOT PLACE CLOTH *INSIDE* BIG OPEN CUTS OR BIG OPEN WOUNDS!** *Bacteria can grow on the tiny plant pieces!* ☹

BONUS: MAKE A NATURAL PAIN RUB
You can make an anti-pain rub using pain herbs. The beeswax will thicken the oil so that it becomes harder.
- Get the herbs and beeswax from your health food store
- Heat two tablespoons of the herb(s) into 4 ounces/125mL of olive or some other healthy oil
- Heat herbs and oil on low heat until it boils
- Once mixture boils turn off heat and strain/remove the herbs
- Add in 10-15 pellets (grain of rice size) of beeswax. **Note**: that beeswax can come in many size pellets (even smaller than a grain of rice) so this is not exact. Let the liquid cool to almost room temperature and if you have put in enough beeswax then your herb formula will have a harder consistency like VaporRub.
- If it is not hard enough yet, reheat the mixture for a few minutes and add in more beeswax. Allow to cool again to nearly room temperature.

- Keep repeating this process until you get the consistency/hardness you want. If you added TOO much beeswax, the mix will be very hard. If you want to soften it then add more oil to the beeswax herb mix and reheat.
- After that you can put your herb formula into a little jar (you can also buy these at the herbal store) or a little bowl and use it. ☺

By the way, you can make ANY rub for ANY purpose this way! I make one of my own hair products by using hair herbs, oil and beeswax! First, I put the herbs and oil into a mason jar. Second, I put that jar under a box and then place the box in a sunny area for a week or two. We call the process of using the sun as a heat source to pull out good parts from the plant a *solar infusion*. Lastly, I add in the beeswax and heat the entire mixture on the stove to get my herb mix to harden. However, in the winter when there is less sun I use the complete stove heating process. I have also made an anti-itch rub and an anti-inflammatory rub like this!

Thanks to JdW for the suggestion of putting in my favorite home herbs!

LOCAL HEALTH FOOD STORES LIST

There are more stores than these but I frequent these the most often and like their variety of herbs and the quality of their merchandise. If you do not live in the Atlanta area very sorry, you will have to find your herbs on your own. However, if you are passing through you can use this list! Keep in mind that store hours or locations can change so please check the website or call prior to making a trip.

RULE: Roots, Berries or Leaves are preferred over powdered herbs

HEALTH FOOD STORES: Atlanta area and suburbs

Downtown
- **Whole Foods Market**—wholefoodsmarket.com/**404.853.1681**/at 650 Ponce de Leon Ave NE, Atlanta, GA 30308/Open daily 730a-10p.

East Side
- **Sevananda**—www.sevanada.coop/**404.681.2831**/at 467 Moreland Avenue NE Atlanta, GA 30307/Open daily 8a-10p.
- **Dekalb Farmer's Market**—www.dekalbfarmersmarket.com/ **404.377.6400**/at 3000 East Ponce De Leon Avenue, Decatur, GA 30033/Open daily 9a-9p.

North Side

- **Health Unlimited**-www.healthunlimitedatlanta.com/**404.633.6677**
  at 2968 North Druid Hills Rd NE, Atlanta, GA 30329/Open Mon-Sat 10a-6p,
  Sun 12-6p

South Side

- **SPN Herbs**-*(my office)* www.spnherbshoppe.com/**770.507.2555**
  at 123 East Atlanta Rd, Stockbridge, GA 30281/Open Mon, Tues, Thurs and
  Friday 10a-7p. Wed 10a-6p. Sat 11a-5p. CLOSED Sun.
- **Herbal Planet**—www.myherbalplanet.com/**678.432.9110**/at 2560 Hwy 42
  North, McDonough, GA 30253/Open Mon-Fri 10a-7p, Sat 10a-6p,
  CLOSED Sun.

WHAT DOES DR. MEGAN DO WHEN SHE IS SICK?

I may catch a cold or flu once every other year. It is perfectly reasonable though to
get a cold/flu/stomach infection once or twice a year. That is healthy because it
keeps your immune system/police on alert. Your body should be able to fight off a
cold within 1-3 days and the flu within a week. If it takes longer than that, you are
severely low in immunity/police force. You often ask me what I do when I am sick
so here are my favorite therapies for myself!

INFECTIONS: Cold, Flu, Diarrhea (food poisoning)

Nutrition

- **I reduce eating**: I eat only one small meal—or I do not eat at all--and I focus
  instead on getting in fluids—*fluids are fast to digest so that we do not use
  energy on digestion and instead all energy goes towards fighting germs and
  healing.*
- **NO SUGAR in ANY form:** no sweets, but also no Bread, Potatoes, Rice,
  Cereals, Pasta, juice and little to no fruit—*sugar slows down healing.*
- **I make soups or a light stir-fry** with green veggies: Broccoli, Mustard
  greens and ½ cup of beans—*a light meal that does not pull away too much
  energy from healing.*
- **Smoothies:** I may use ½ a Banana, Avocado then Cinnamon, Nutmeg,
  Ginger powder, sliced Almonds and Kale--*again easy to make, very light put
  packed full of germ fighting stuff!*
- **Avocado**: I might eat it alone with salt or in a smoothie or soup--*packed
  with vitamins for healing!*
- **I add anti-germ** herbs to my food such as Garlic, Onions, Oregano,
  Cinnamon, Sage and Ginger.
- **Cayenne pepper:** this is a driver herb meaning it helps the other herbs get
  to where they need to go (like a bus or taxi driver takes you where you

need to go) so I put a little of the powdered cayenne in with food. The liquid cayenne I add a few drops into my teas. Of course, I only use cayenne from Dr. Shulze[4] because his brand is the purest and strongest in my opinion.

Fluids

- **I drink half of my body weight in water**—*water helps us get rid of trash that makes us sick via the main organs of elimination/trash removal systems.*
- **Thyme and Rosemary tea**. Three tablespoons of each herb in 4 cups/1 Liter of water. Bring to boil. Turn off fire. *I usually do a quick steam inhalation treatment right there!* ☺ Then I add the juice of one fresh squeezed lemon or lime and a teaspoon of raw, local honey. I drink 2 cups/16 ounces/500 mL in the morning and in the evening…or all day long if I am very sick. This is my <u>FAVORITE</u> "I am sick drink"! ☺
- **Other teas**: I may make Ginger root, Oregano or Sage tea or sometimes I will put all these herbs into the Thyme and Rosemary tea!
- **Garlic "shots"**: I cut up finely (or pass through a garlic press) 2-3 big cloves of Garlic. Then I put the Garlic in ¼ cup/63 mL of Orange juice or Apple juice and I chew the Garlic a little bit and then swallow down the mixture! You can use any juice---Garlic is VERY strongly anti-microbial so it kills viruses, bacteria and fungi! I may take 3-4 shots a day. Or sometimes I will actually make the Garlic drink I mentioned earlier. *Bad breath.* ☹ *Good health.* ☺
  Note: with kids you can make a Garlic "melt" by using 1-2 cloves of Garlic in 1 teaspoon of honey. Let them chew well and swallow! *Raw honey is best.*
- **No drinking of cold fluids/out of the fridge or with ice**: drinking cold beverages makes the body pull energy away from fighting germs/healing in order to heat up the drink to a temperature the body prefers. ALL drinks are room temperature or warmed. EVEN WATER is heated!

Supplements

I take my usual daily supplements-Fish oil, Multivitamin/Mineral, Probiotic, Vitamin D-however I typically double the doses. Additionally I may take these:

- **Priority One brand BioVegetarian**—I take two tablets every two hours for the first day I am sick, then two tablets every four hours for the other days. *This is a natural antibiotic! It is super powerful because it is jam packed with vitamins and minerals needed for healing. It also has all of the major germ fighting herbs such as Echinacea, Myrrh, Ginger, Garlic, Cayenne, Oregon Grape Root, Barberry.* This tablet tastes totally disgusting.☹ I mean just the smell ALONE is frightful and could scare away a germ but the taste is even worse! I am <u>VERY </u>used to taking bad tasting herbs because that is all

221

we used in my household growing up! We did not use even a Tylenol for illness. No antibiotics. I never even knew that medicine was "in a pill form" or that they come in orange or white bottles because all of our medicines were always teas from fresh plants (out of the garden) that were green or brown or a store bought syrup that was made from a plant.

Therefore when I say that this tablet is nasty tasting I do not exaggerate! This tablet is REALLY powerful though! I do not think ANY germ can fight back against it! ☺ I have a hard time getting it down but I do it! It is also hard for me because it is a tablet and very big and I was never good with swallowing supplements which is why I usually take supplements with food. I chew the food first and then just before I swallow I throw the supplement in my mouth and everything goes down smoothly. Tablets are not as smooth as capsules and so I struggle with it for that reason too. But I take the BioVeg with a meal or a piece of food and I can swallow it that way. **WARNING: if you are pregnant/trying to become pregnant/or could get pregnant "by accident" you should not take this.** It contains 10,000 IU of Vitamin A in just two tablets and Vitamin A at doses higher than 10,000 IU can cause serious birth defects in an unborn baby! ☹

- **NewMark brand Immune Defense**—if I cannot get the Bio Veg--because around the cold season, it is hard to keep it in stock--I will use this. It has a blend of medicinal mushrooms, which are great for strengthening the immune system/police. It has Reishi, Shitake, Maitake, Cordyceps and more!—I take 2 capsules every three hours or so. If I am very sick, I will take 2 capsules every hour.
- **Gaia Herbs brand Black Elderberry Syrup**—Elderberry (Sambucus nigra in Latin) is a fantastic herb for fighting viruses and infection especially if there is a slight fever. It does not "turn off" your fever alarm but instead helps your body fight! I really LOVE the taste of this syrup and have to stop myself from taking it even when I am not sick, so I do not buy it too often but it is great especially for kids! I probably take one or two teaspoons at night only before bed.

- **Other great sickness supplements are Vitamin C, Vitamin E, and Zinc.** If I use Vitamin C, alone it is in the ascorbate form and I use the pure powder (unsweetened) and put about a tablespoon or so of it into some orange juice a few times a day. Since commercial Vitamin C often has ADDED sugar into it (bad) when you taste the true Vitamin C powder that is unsweetened, it is so sour it will make your face twist like a pretzel! ☺

Home therapies

When I am sick, I also do therapies at home to help the body to heal.

- **Castor Oil Cloth/pack:** I sleep with it on my stomach/low abdomen to help stimulate my immune system to work better! If I have a cough or chest congestion then I will sleep with it on my chest and or back. *Sometimes I soak two cloths and wear one on my back and chest and abdomen and then wrap myself with Saran wrap and sleep with them that way!*

- **Chest rub:** If I am coughing a lot, I will rub my chest with Aboniki Balm and then put a towel under my shirt and sleep with it overnight. The Aboniki has peppermint in it that helps calm down a crazy cough and helps you breathe better. The towel helps keep the chest muscles warm, which also stops them from contracting as often and making you cough. If I do not have Aboniki then I will use Vicks VapoRub. However, Aboniki is much better! You can find it online or you can get it from African, Caribbean or Asian Stores.
  *Thanks mama VO for introducing it to me!

- **Sunshine and fresh air:** I sit by the window and let the sun shine on me—*the sun has healing properties and fresh air cleans out the lungs.* I do this even if it is cold and I have to dress up like an Eskimo. I may not open the window entirely but just open it half way or a crack. **Note:** the **sun** has gotten **a bad reputation** these last few years as being **a big, yellow, evil ball in the sky** that causes skin cancer **and that is not true.** Instead of blaming the sun for your skin cancer, you should look into your lifestyle and see why your body was not able to kill cancer cells that may have developed. Although it is true that it is not a good idea to be in the sun all day. Particularly during the hottest part of the day, until your skin turns red like a lobster or purple like an eggplant. Avoid the hottest hours of sunlight especially if it is not for work reasons but instead only to get a tan.☹

- **A short walk:** perhaps only 10 minutes or so. *It helps to move blood/semi-trucks around the body and they remove trash and bring helpful germ fighting nutrients!*

- **Steam Inhalation Treatment:** if I have nasal or chest congestion/difficulty breathing/cough/mucus/phlegm. Once or twice a day.

- **Rest:** I make sure I go to bed early and even reschedule appointments. I sit on the couch and watch nature shows on TV and other programs I like. Keep in mind that even though you take natural supplements and do natural treatments, one of Nature's 9 Health Laws is SLEEP/REST! Therefore, try to take off work! Even if you can only afford to take one day or a half-day that is better than nothing! Or if it is possible to work from home try that. But if you can afford to take off from work financially speaking, then do so! Otherwise, even doing all these great therapies you STILL may not get well!

- **I stay away from kids:** they are loveable, germ carrying balls of energy! They usually love to share things _especially_ germs so I stay away from babies and little kids 12 or under. And other sick adults.
- **Dr. Shulze[4] Air Detox:** it has essential oils of Eucalyptus-a strong lung herb, Grapefruit, Lime, Lemon and Orange. I spray it in the main room I am sitting in and it helps to clean the air! It smells so good that it lifts my spirits! Usually when I am sick, the smell of mucus, cough, diarrhea and fluffing (farting) is so annoying that it is nice to smell something fresh! ☺

OTHER HEALTH ISSUES I MAY GET

Again, I am not frequently ill but on occasion I get other little annoying things and so I will just mention them here:

- **Ear infection: Herb Pharm brand Mullein Garlic Pure Ear Oil.** I put a few drops into my ear every hour. The Garlic kills bad "bugs" and Mullein is an herb that helps with pain (analgesic) and healing and inflammation.
  Note: it is always a good idea to get an ear infection/ear pain or fluid coming out of your ear checked out by a health professional before putting anything into the ear. If there is a bad enough infection you may have a hole in your eardrum, which is at the end of your ear tunnel inside your ear. If you have a hole in your eardrum then you should not put drops of ANYTHING into the ear. However, if you already had it checked and you know that you do not have a hole in your eardrum it is ok to use drops.

- **Eye infection:** like pink eye (conjunctivitis). I usually just get it in one eye, especially the right eye. I will often get this if I do not wash my hands well and then I rub my eyes. My eyes NEVER turn pink or red though, instead my eye will be leaking clear fluid all day long or sometimes just a few times a day. Other times I may see a big ball of yellow goop in my eye (goop is a medical term...just kidding it really is not) and since I do not have "goopy" eyes then I know I am about to get an infection there. Sometimes I can wake up with my eyelids stuck together if the eye was "leaking" overnight and then I cannot open my eye without washing it with warm water first.
  (1)Herb Pharm brand Rue Fennel for external use. 10 drops in a glass eye wash cup full of room temperature water. I buy the glass eye wash cup at a pharmacy like CVS/Walgreens or at a health food store. **Note:** It is very important not to put dirty water into the eyes OR nose-like if you use a Neti pot for your sinuses! So first, I boil distilled or alkaline water and then let it cool down to room temperature. I also boil the glass eyecup for 5-10 minutes to kill anything that may be on the cup. I wash the sick eye at least 5-6 times in the day. I also wash the non-sick eye 2-3 times just because

sometimes since the virus or bacteria is being "chased" out of the sick eye it will try to crawl into the non-sick eye and infect that one! **(2)** If I do not have Rue Fennel external use formula then I use **fresh Lemon or Lime in water**. I squeeze half of the Lemon or Lime and <u>put only ¼</u> of the juice into a clean, boiled, glass eye wash cup. I rinse both eyes at least 5 times/day. *If it is a very strong bacteria or virus and it is putting up a fight, I may use both of the eye wash recipes and simply alternate between them!*

Question: Doesn't Lemon sting your eyes like crazy you ask? YES! I actually see "stars" like on the cartoons when someone is dizzy. However, Lemon helps clean out the eye and bring blood to the eye! Therefore, I am not a pansy (coward) with this treatment! Feel the burn! ☺

Note: A more convenient (and less messy) way to wash out the eye is to use a 2 ounce dropper bottle to treat the eyes. You can buy them at a health food store or medical store. Then you just fill up the dropper bottle(s) with either the ¼ Lemon or Lime fresh juice and the boiled water (now cooled down) OR the 20 drops of Rue Fennel external use herb formula with the boiled water (now cooled down). I shake the bottle(s) well before every use and drop 3-4 drops of the mix into each eye at least 5-10 times in the day. I dose almost every hour. Using a dropper bottle makes it easy to carry my eye treatments wherever I go!
Do not touch the tip of the dropper tube to your eye or to anything else!

- **Sore throat**—I will make Thyme and Rosemary tea and then gargle the back of my throat with it. If the back of my throat has mucus, I will gargle and spit out the tea and then I may actually drink the next mouthful!
I often buy a bottle of throat cough spray, empty the liquid and wash it well. Then I put my anti-bug herb tea (room temperature) into the spray bottle and spray the back of my throat with the herb tea all day. It is easy to carry along wherever. I leave it out of the fridge at room temp.

If I am only a little sick I may only do one or two of all my suggestions.
If I am very sick, I do a few of them. At minimum, I do Thyme and Rosemary tea, water, avoiding sugar, steam inhalation, Castor Oil cloth and rest.
I do this until the symptoms go away and then TWO days after that. Sometimes the germs are dying off but if you stop treating too early they get some extra energy and try to take over the body again, so that is why we continue a few days past when the symptoms stop. **You can do this!**

Chapter 16: Natural Products for your Home and Body

It is important to know how many toxins/bad chemicals are in the environment. They are literally EVERYWHERE from makeup, soap, plastic cups to the vinyl in our shower curtains to the paint on the walls and the colors/dyes in our clothes! For example, some air fresheners and mothballs contain Para-dichlorobenzene which can cause immediate symptoms such as fatigue, headache, nausea, and vomiting and with long term high exposure serious problems in Skin, Liver and Brain cities![25]

If you really want to **get an in depth look into just how polluted our environment** is you can read a book called Our Toxic World: A Wake Up Call.[26] You can also keep up to date on toxins in our food and environment and how to avoid them on the Environmental Working Group's website www.ewg.org.[27]

Since we cannot avoid ALL bad chemicals from all sources, the idea is to !limit the amount of toxic things we expose ourselves to little by little. We can especially be successful with products we use every day on our body and around the house. You do not need to change everything at once. Just pick one thing and then start adding on. I just stopped using the $1 dollar deodorant and changed to a less toxic deodorant that costs about $6 so it is not much more expensive but since I use deodorant every day (multiple times a day if I am really smelly ☹) now I know I have reduced another source of bad chemicals on my skin. ☺

COMMON TOXIC CHEMICALS
There are some especially bad chemicals that have been linked to possibly causing cancer to develop so try to avoid/lower exposure in your personal body products and or around the house:

- **Bisphenol A (BPA)**—chemical used to make plastics for food and beverage containers and the lining of food and beverage cans. *Limit: using plastic containers (especially freezing or microwaving food in them!). Limit canned foods.*
- **Atrazine**—an herbicide/weed killer. Found in drinking water. *Limit:* by using *water filters.*
- **Organophosphate Pesticides**—insecticides/bug killers. *Limit: by buying organic produce when possible (or wash really well with a great soap); use less produce with the highest amount of pesticides on them called the "Dirty Dozen".* These usually are fruits with thin skins like apples etc. See more about the "Dirty Dozen on the EWG website. www.ewg.org.[27]

- **Phthalates**—used in makeup/cosmetics, soft and flexible plastics like shower curtains and plastic toys, aerosol sprays (like air fresheners), food wraps and rain coats. *Limit:* these are hard to avoid! *Use an umbrella instead of raincoat? Just kidding!* ☺ *Use quality cosmetics with the least amount of chemicals possible. Use essential oils instead of air fresheners. Limit storing food in plastics. Use glass. Avoid products with the word "fragrance" in it.*
- **Lead**—found in drinking water, old paints and in other countries in gasoline. *Limit: by using water filters and buy quality paints and take care when removing paint from the walls.*
- **Mercury**—high amount in seafood and especially farmed fish. *Limit: by avoiding fish grown on farms instead of caught out in the wild. A good brand of wild caught fish is Wild Alaskan Salmon.*
- **PFCs (Per or Polyfluorochemicals)**—used to make water, grease and stain repellant coatings. *Limit: home applied carpet and furniture treatments, fast food and greasy carryout foods, microwaveable popcorn bags, and personal products without PTFE or fluoro ingredients.*
- **Triclosan**—used in many liquid hand and dishwashing soaps as well as personal care products. *Limit: just do not wash dishes! YAY!* ☺ *Ok maybe not...instead try to look for soaps without it.* Avoid especially the anti-bacterial soaps.
- **Nonylphenol**—used widely in detergents, paints, personal care products and plastics. *Limit: avoid/decrease use of products with this ingredient in it.*

BODY PRODUCTS

It can be difficult to find a product with NO bad chemicals at all in it so just do your best to find one that has the LEAST amount of bad chemicals.

In general, it is best to avoid/limit these in any product you use on your body: Sulfates, Parabens, Phthalates, Propylene Glycol, Mineral Oil, synthetic/fake Fragrances, and synthetic colors.

The main items we use daily are soaps, lotions, hair products, shaving cream, facial products including makeup, toothpaste and deodorant.
Many of the brands I listed carry an entire line that covers all of these areas.

There are many good personal care brands out there; I just included a few here. You can use them as a guide to find a brand that is similar if these are not available in your local health food store. You can also order from an online health food store like Vitacost.com, Amazon or even on their individual websites.

- Alaffia   www.alaffia.com
- Avalon Organics   www.avalonorganics.com
- JASON   www.jason-personalcare.com
- Nature's Gate   www.naturesgate.com
- Desert Essence   www.desertessence.com
- Suki   www.sukiskincare.com
- DeVita   www.devitaskincare.com
- Super Salve Company   www.supersalve.com
- Nelson's Natural World   www.nelsonsnaturalworld.com
- J.R. Watkins Apothecary   www.jrwatkins.com
- Alba Botanica   www.albabotanica.com

Many thanks to Dr. Flynn[28] and Dr. Roberson[29] for their valuable contributions on skin care and cosmetic products! They are natural skin and hair gurus!

DR. MEGAN'S FAVORITE BODY PRODUCTS!
What I use myself to try to be as natural as possible. ☺

HAIR
Shea Moisture brand—shampoo/conditioners and anti-breakage masque.

MAKEUP
I only wear lipstick/lip gloss and I use Mary Kay for the lipstick and a cheap shiny lip-gloss.☹ I have a hard time spending $20 on a tube of lipstick (so I do not) but there are some great companies with fantastic products that do not have lead, bat poop (yes, the flying mammals) or other gross stuff in their products. Of course, that makes their products a little more expensive. I am working my way up to the expensive lip gloss. ☺ But if I did wear more makeup, I would use the two below.

- Arbonne
- Jane Iredale

TOOTHPASTE
Nature's Gate brand Peppermint

DEODORANT
J. R. Watkins Apothecary brand Aloe and Green Tea.

Note: there are many kinds of natural deodorants like the deodorant rocks etc. It is VERY important to remember that since they are non-toxic *you may need to reapply* more than once in the day. *If you walk by and you are killing plants and wildlife with your body odor then that is not good.*☹ Experiment with many natural deodorants to see if they are strong enough for you.
If they do not work as well as a more toxic deodorant, then **PLEASE do humankind a favor**, keep your toxic deodorant and work on detoxing/eliminating a bad chemical from *somewhere else* in your life.☺

SOAP
Vitamin E bar of soap—*only has Vitamin E and Glycerin*

SKIN MOISTURIZERS
- **J.R. Watkins Apothecary brand Lemon Cream Lotion**—for light moisture
  It smells so good, I seriously wish I could eat it! ☺☺
- **Almond oil**—for medium moisture
- **Shea Butter**—for heavy moisture like in the winter or before swimming in a pool.

I must confess that I am actually very bad about putting on lotions and or creams...especially on my feet.☹ *It is funny because when my brother A comes to visit from another state he will often ask me "Megan, don't they sell lotion in Georgia?!?" My inner circle will periodically inspect my feet like my sister G and or my mom and will say "Oh, they don't look so bad today" or if they do look bad then they just shake their heads. I am improving slowly in this area though.* ☺

SHOWER FILTERS
When I lived in Arizona, every time I turned on the water I could smell Chlorine. I felt like I was at the pool! My skin would be SO dry and cracked after the shower that I looked like an old lizard.☹ I decided to buy a shower filter and I was human again!
- You can buy them from big stores like Walmart, Home Depot/Lowes. That way if it does not fit your shower head you can easily return it
- Nikken Brand PiMag Micro Jet Shower System[22]

HOUSE HOLD PRODUCTS

What we use around the house on a day-to-day basis can also be toxic so try to reduce the bad chemicals by using some of these brands.

CLEANERS AND DETERGEANTS (for dishes and laundry)
- Seventh Generation
- Sun and Earth
- Planet 2X

You can also visit the Environmental Working Group[27] website for their Guide to Healthy Cleaning.

DR. MEGAN'S FAVORITE HOUSEHOLD PRODUCTS!
The things I use!

AIR FRESHENERS
Dr. Schulze's Air Detox[4]

ESSENTIAL OILS
You can put these in small water fountains around the house and the constant recycling of the water in the fountain will spread the essential oils aroma completely and make your home smell great!

- Nature's Alchemy brand
- Now brand

CLEANERS
- **White vinegar**—I use it in a spray bottle to spray down all hard surfaces like kitchen and bathroom countertops!
- **Baking soda and soap**—the baking soda is abrasive/scratchy and with the soap, the two are a perfect combination for cleaning bathtubs and sinks!

Note: these two options are MUCH less toxic than bleach. ☺ On occasion, I do still use bleach for things but I use *very* small amounts and open the windows!

SUMMER TIME and OUTSIDE USE PRODUCTS
- Burt's Bees brand
- Many of the brands under body products also have outside use/summertime products!

INSECT SPRAY ESSENTIAL OIL RECIPE

Again, these are products to have around the house anyway just because they can be used for many different things! The Apple Cider Vinegar helps Digestion city work better, Jojoba oil is great for skin and hair, Eucalyptus oil is fantastic to inhale for any problem in and relating to Lung city (sinus/chest congestion, asthma etc.), Clove oil is used topically/on surface for tooth pain and Lemon grass is great for rubbing over achy joints with arthritis!

- 1 cup/250mL purified Water
- 1/cup/125mL unfiltered Apple Cider Vinegar
- ½ cup/125mL Jojoba oil

20 drops of each essential oil:

- Lemongrass oil
- Citronella oil
- Eucalyptus oil
- Lemon oil
- Clove oil

Mix all ingredients (and store) in a glass bottle and then pour some of the mixture into a spray bottle and it is ready! Shake before each use.

Too lazy/not enough time to make a natural bug product? That is ok! You can purchase Dr. Shulze[4] Bug Block spray or Bug Barrier cream!

MORE HERBS THAT INSECTS HATE

The herbs above are easy to find while these may be a little harder to find but I still want you to have this list. You can sprinkle a few drops outside the house around garage doors and regular doors as well as put a few drops inside the house around doors/windows to keep ants and other insects from taking over your house. You may need to use a lot more than a few drops if you have a big insect problem, or you may have to reapply outside if it rains. Another way to apply the essential oils to a problem area is by putting 5-10 drops onto a cotton ball and then wiping the area with it.

- Sandalwood
- Geranium
- Camphor
- Patchouli
- Penny Royal

- Rosewood
- Atlas Cedar

Thanks to E Thorne for the extra insect herbs list!

NATURAL SUNSCREEN RECIPE

The ingredients may cost more up front than buying a regular cheaper sunscreen but the recipe will last for a long time. In addition, you can use these oils around the house for other things such as the Coconut oil on hair or as a makeup remover, the Avocado oil on salads/for cooking and the Almond oil on skin! Mix all ingredients well in a small bowl and then pour into a spray bottle and use!
This recipe is an SPF sun protection of about 30 and you need to remember to shake before each use and reapply a few times in the day.

- ½ cup/125mL of Coconut oil
- ½ cup/125mL of Avocado oil
- 50 drops of Carrot Seed oil
- 20 drops of Almond oil

CHAPTER 17: Got Supplements? Which ones you *REALLY* need and why!

Many people are taking at least one to three prescription medications. However, in the last few years, there has been an explosive interest in taking natural supplements. So I thought I would help you understand how supplements tidy up your health, what to look for in a supplement and which ones you actually NEED.

WHY DO WE USE SUPPLEMENTS ANYWAY?

Well that is because of four main reasons **(1)** we are mass-producing food and **over farming** the land that we grow food on. We do not let the farm land rest, so that it can replenish the minerals and helpful stuff in the soil. Therefore, the soil is not as full of minerals as it used to be years ago, which means that the food grown in the ground does not contain the same amount of vitamins and minerals that it did years ago. Even if we are eating a healthy diet, our food still does not contain enough healthy nutrients. **(2)** There is a lot of food that was NEVER grown in mother Earth but instead this "food" **was made in a lab.** *That is a problem in and of itself!* They often use many colors and preservatives to give the food a longer shelf life so that the cereal you just bought can last on your shelf for a year! *That is bad in case you are wondering.* The colors and additives or processing and packaging of foods also removes many of the helpful vitamins and minerals.
(3) We often **over cook food** and thereby kill/destroy all the helpful vitamins they contain. No, broccoli should never melt in your mouth; you should have to chew it!

      Analogy*: what happens to you after you spend too much time in a hot tub? Your hands and feet become wrinkly and prune-y right? So what do you do when you see that? You get out of the hot tub right? Well the same thing happens when we over cook vegetables. Especially the green ones such as Kale, Spinach, and Collard greens. Green veggies are full of B Vitamins, which are very heat sensitive, so once the greens reach a certain temperature they change color and you know they are getting too hot/wrinkly. But if you keep cooking them the greens do not get out of the pot/hot tub. Why not? They have no legs!* ☹ So instead, all of the useful heat sensitive B vitamins are <u>cooked to death</u> (literally) and you now just spent energy to make and eat something that might taste very nice but will not help your body with anything at all. In fact, it will take energy away from your body! ☹ ☹ **(4)** We are **unable to make** a necessary nutrient in our body or make *enough of it*. For example, humans cannot make Vitamin C in our bodies--other animals can--so we must eat it or supplement this because we need Vitamin C to help heal skin and fight infection. Other nutrients we do not make at all are the mineral Iron, Vitamin B12, and Essential Fatty Acids/Omega 3s (EPA/DHA).

DO NOT OVER "DRUG" YOURSELF WITH A TON OF SUPPLEMENTS EITHER!

While it is true that supplements in general are not harming your body the way a prescription/over the counter medication is, it is *still* not good to be taking twelve supplements instead of taking twelve medications! *Gasp!* What in the world do you mean Dr. Megan? Thank you for asking, I will tell you! What I mean is that your goal should ALWAYS be to get back in tune with Nature's 9 Health Laws. In this case, with respect to nutrition, make sure you are choosing healthy foods and cooking them properly and that you are not using too many supplements as an excuse to keep eating a poor diet. Again, we cannot break Nature's 9 and then try to balance it with prescribed drugs OR natural supplements!

WHAT SUPPLEMENTS DO I REALLY NEED?

Usually the three basic supplements needed in the United States of You to be able to work well are a multivitamin, probiotic, and fish oil/essential fatty acid (EFA). However, a person may need one or two more depending on the specific illness they are working to heal themselves of. For example, a person with osteoporosis/bone loss may decide to add a specific supplement that adds specific nutrients that help bones rebuild. As for dosing, I do not touch on that here since again, that is individual depending on what type of illness a person has. A person who has high blood pressure will not take the same doses of tea(s) or supplement(s) as a person who is helping their body heal itself of cancer. The person with high blood pressure may need more or vice versa.

WHAT SHOULD I LOOK FOR IN A SUPPLEMENT?

Two things are the most important and that is quality and quantity. You want to avoid supplements that are **(1) poor in quality** meaning that the constituents were either over processed (dead) or contain harmful elements. Things such as sugar, or colors. Some supplements contain human body parts! Other supplements are not in the best form for the body to use. **(2) poor in quantity** meaning that the amounts of the constituents are not enough to affect the body to any measurable degree. *Analogy: That is like if I were to tell you I had not eaten in three days, and so you say, "wait Dr. Megan, I will get you some food!" You run away, come back, and give me only two saltine crackers! I would be super angry with you because two crackers will not do ANYTHING to help my hunger after three days of not eating! This is true with many supplements there just is not enough product in there to help a HEALTHY person, much less a VERY SICK PERSON!*

HOW DO I PICK A BRAND?

There are many supplement companies but the majority of their products do not work or are even dangerous because they are either poor in quality and or poor in quantity. Now you are **wasting your HARD EARNED money** on a product that *at best* may not help you, or *at WORST* may hurt you! Therefore, we naturopathic doctors promote usage of physician grade supplements from nutraceutical or natural vitamin companies that we trust. We routinely and randomly investigated them. Yes! That means we have sent sneaky investigators to research how these companies find, grow, make, store and ship their natural supplements and we have found these companies to provide consistent results in quality and quantity. Generally speaking though, if you bought a supplement in a gas station, a Walmart or at the mall, then more than likely I would be suspicious of it. Sometimes they can be ok, but usually it is rubbish. ☹

Therefore, if your supplement brand does not appear on this list we are uncertain of its safety and efficacy and will not likely endorse it.

This list is not complete but does represent the major brands that we use most often and are in the highest tier or tier 1 of supplements available to help your body restore health! My favorite brands are **bolded** ☺:

- Allergy Research Group
- Ayush Herbs
- Bach Flower Remedies
- DaVinci Labs
- **Designs for Health**
- **Gaia Herbs**
- Heel/BHI
- **Herb Pharm**
- Hyland Homeopathics
- Innate
- Integrative Therapeutics
- **Klaire Labs**
- Nordic Naturals
- **Perque**
- **Pharmax**
- Priority One
- ProThera
- Pure Encapsulations
- **Seroyal/Genestra**
- Standard Process
- Thorne

- Vital Nutrients
- **Wise Woman Herbals**

Most of these brands are not sold in regular stores like Walmart or GNC. Some health food stores such as Wholefoods may carry a few products from these brands.
Look locally or you can also order through your friendly neighborhood naturopathic physician or order online. However, another reputable company that I love and whom you can order from directly that offer 2nd tier quality supplements would be
Life Extension.[35]

DR. MEGAN'S FAVORITE SUPPLEMENT BRANDS
I periodically research new supplements but for right now these are my favorites that I even use myself:

- **Multivitamin/mineral**--Klaire Labs brand Vitaspectrum capsule formula **OR** Dr Shulze[4] Superfood Plus (powder or tablets)
  Vitamins and minerals are needed for energy and all basic body function!
- **Probiotic**--Genestra brand HMF Intensive
  Healthy bacteria for digestion and immune function!
- **Fish oil**--Genestra brand Super EFA liquid orange flavor
  Important for the brain, building body parts and healing!

Those who will not use fish oil-such as vegans or people with fish allergies-can use flaxseed oil to try to get their EFA/essential fatty acids/Omega 3's.

- **Flaxseed oil**—Genestra brand Organic Vegan EFA liquid pineapple flavor

Note: You need certain enzymes to convert flaxseed into the essential fatty acid. Many people lack these enzymes. Therefore, if you lack these enzymes you could be taking a product that your body may or may not be able to use. For that reason, we typically prefer people to use fish oil if they do not have a true fish allergy.
The body can easily use fish oil without a problem in MOST people.

Some additional supplements that I may use are protein powder, Glutamine, Vitamin B12, Vitamin C, Vitamin D, Magnesium and Calcium/Magnesium and Iron. Glutamine is an amino acid that "feeds" the healthy bacteria in Digestion city. Therefore because Glutamine is feeding the bacteria it is what we call a "prebiotic". *Analogy: so if YOU were bacteria (a probiotic) and I gave you a sandwich to eat, the sandwich would be the prebiotic*. Vitamin D is used in hundreds of areas in the body and actually in some cases can act like a hormone/mail carrier and not just like a vitamin and most people are low in this. Iron is a mineral that people are often VERY low in especially growing children and women because of bleeding too much with their menses/periods or in pregnancy.

Analogy: Think of a semi-truck that is delivering oranges from the state of Florida to the state of Georgia. Your red blood cells/semi-trucks carry boxes called Hemoglobin and inside those Hemoglobin boxes would be the Iron. You can think of the iron as being the oranges! **Quick Note on Iron:** it is very possible to have normal iron levels in your blood work but that your body is not using iron well so be sure if you have fatigue or low energy to ask/remind your doctor to do an IRON PANEL, which will also check how you are USING iron. Do not assume that an iron panel was done because sadly <u>very often</u> it is not ordered, as it should be.

Iron Analogy: this would be like if you bought a box of oranges (iron) from the grocery store but then left the box in the garage. Technically, you have enough oranges (iron) because they are in your garage but since you do not have them in the kitchen you are not using them properly. Make sense?

- **Protein Powder**—Designs for Health brand Pure Pea Natural Vanilla flavor or unsweetened flavor
- **Prebiotic**—Designs for Health brand L-Glutamine 850mg
- **Vitamin B12**---Perque brand Activated B12 Guard 2000mcg lozenges
- **Vitamin C**---Dr Shulze[4] Super C-Plus OR Perque brand Potent C Guard. *These two are the best quality therefore more expensive. A second tier supplement is from Life Extension[35] brand Fast-C. Still better than what they sell in most stores!*
- **Vitamin D**—Genestra brand D Mulsion 1000 IU liquid drops
- **Iron**—Perque brand Hematin **OR** Integrative Therapeutics brand Liquid Iron Cinnamon flavor **OR** Vitanica brand Iron Extra (capsules) **OR** DaVinci Laboratories Bis-Glycinate (capsules).
- **Magnesium**---Perque brand Mg Plus Guard
- **Calcium and Magnesium**---Perque brand Bone Guard Forté 20

WARNING: Iron can poison children so keep iron supplements well out of reach of little hands! Really, keep all supplements, medicines, cleaning supplies and ANYTHING else in a jar, bag or spray bottle away from kids. Use child locks or rubber bands on low cabinets or better yet store these items in high cabinets.

Another note on Iron: For Stomach city to break iron apart properly, you need enough stomach acid. Therefore, if you are low in stomach acid you can take all the iron supplements or prescribed iron that you want but your body cannot use it. Additionally, Vitamin C helps the body to use iron. Hence, it is not a bad idea to take your iron with dark leafy greens since they actually have more Vitamin C than oranges/citrus. However, if you really want to you can take your iron with Orange juice☺. You will find that most natural iron supplements will have Vitamin C in the bottle as well…for this very reason. The dosing of Iron in natural supplements is VERY different from the dosing in prescription Iron; as are the Iron forms themselves. For this reason, you need to work with an informed health professional.
In case you forgot, you can do this!

CHAPTER 18: I think I can do this! What is the secret to success?

The best strategy for success is to study this book very well for a few days, mentally and physically prepare yourself and your household to make adjustments—like if you have to finish eating or throw out unhealthy foods. Get a support system in place, at least one person that will help your journey to health. Remember, it may not necessarily be a spouse/partner, close friend or family member so keep in mind friends at school, coworkers, religious/spiritual buddies ANYONE who can help encourage you and keep you accountable! It is easy to quit on ourselves or to let ourselves down, but it is hard to disappoint someone else who believes in you and is trying to help you, so find that one person! Of course, the more people helping you the better ☺ and then pick a start date to begin tidying up your body and helping it to restore health to itself as it is already able to do!

For optimal health, we have to do all 9, but do not be overwhelmed by everything that you have learned about just now and decide that it is too much. Maybe just start small and pick one thing that you learned about, like drinking enough water for your body weight or avoiding/reducing how much table sugar you take in every day—instead of 3 sodas a day just drink 2! Do not feel overwhelmed and then use that as an excuse to do nothing.

QUESTION: how do you eat an elephant? One bite at a time! Do not try to bite off the entire elephant leg if you feel like it will be too much; instead, start chewing on his toenail. *I bet elephant toenails taste disgusting.* ☹ As you get used to the one change you made, then add on another change and soon you will be doing all of Nature's 9! You will be eating the whole elephant without having to remind yourself...just as you no longer forget to brush your teeth in the morning. Well maybe you do still forget to brush your teeth.☹ Do your best and stay positive. Anything worth having takes effort in the beginning. Even little changes will help the United States of You. Remember, this saying *"A little bit of something, is still better than a whole lot of nothing"!*

SERIOUSLY YOU CAN DO THIS!
You can change your health, just as you change your clothing! Health is not hard or expensive! You can look very nice with clothing from a second hand/thrift store, so start getting healthy and begin styling and profiling! It depends on your choices! Just decide to do it! **Your mind is the ONLY thing holding you back! So change your mind!** Health is a journey! Quick, think of a city or country where you would like to travel to right now...do you have it in your mind? Health is a journey because there are steps that you have to take to get you to that city/country you

want to get to, and every decision that you make or DO NOT make will either take you CLOSER or FARTHER away from your destination.

STORY: I had always wanted to visit Australia. So a few years ago, I finally decided to go. What are the steps I needed to take to get there? First, I needed to save some money (one step closer to Australia). Then I needed to plan what month to leave (one step closer). Then school got busy and my computer stopped working so I had to wait a month to buy my airplane ticket. (a few steps farther away from Australia). Afterwards though, I fixed my computer and then I bought my ticket (closer). Finally, the night before the trip I packed my suitcase (really close) but then UNPACKED a few things I decided that I did not want to take after all. (a tiny step farther away) and the next day I got on the plane and flew there and had a blast! HOORAY I arrived!

Try this: *Stand up right now and walk a few steps in a straight line. Now walk a few steps backwards. Now walk forwards again. Ok, well you do not have to walk if you really do not want to…you can imagine it too.* Likewise with your health, the choices you make DAILY with Nature's 9 Health laws will affect whether you are taking ***steps closer to total health***--like eating well, sleeping on time, drinking water, or if you are taking ***steps farther away from health***--like thinking bad thoughts about yourself or others, not exercising. Now the size of the steps forward or backward depend on HOW MUCH and HOW OFTEN you do a good thing for health or a bad thing against health. **Analogy:** *eating an ENTIRE cake would be like taking ten BIG steps away from health, while just eating a tiny slice of cake would be like taking one small step backwards. Do you understand?* DAILY we want our steps to add up to be MORE steps TOWARDS health, and have fewer steps that lead away from health! As we get more used to being in tune with Nature's 9 Health laws then those steps leading us closer to health become habits and then we do them without having to try or even without thinking about them! Then those habits will become LIFESTYLE! ☺

Think: *when was the last time you left the house without any clothes or shoes on? Not since you were a baby right? Now that it is a habit for you to put on clothes and shoes, you do not even think about it! Except maybe to decide WHAT you want to wear, but you definitely do not forget and go out naked or barefoot though right?* Same with getting in tune with Nature's 9! You will get used to drinking enough water, picking the right foods, paying attention to bedtime, and you will learn to think positively! You CAN get healthy! It is not as if you are trying to travel to the moon. You can arrive at your destination: Health city! So get moving! Even if you do not do ALL 9 at once, pick ONE and just try to do that most of the time then add on the others little by little. **You can do this!** ☺

CHAPTER 19: I am doing Nat's 9 and I am <u>MUCH</u> better but I still need help!

If after two to four months of ACTIVELY and CONSISTENTLY practicing ALL nine of these health laws you do not see the level of improvement you desire, it is possible that your health issue is not a do it yourself (DIY) kind of problem. **Your issue may need a trained eye to locate the specific source of the problem(s).**
It is ok to change your car oil and windshield wiper fluid etc. but when the engine blows up or the breaks fail, you need to take it to a professional mechanic! Likewise, for your health, so once you know you need professional help with your health it would be ideal to:

- **Work with <u>me</u>[24] because I am the best...Ok, I suppose I am biased.** ☺
- However, if that is not possible, other healthcare professionals can help you as well. You may have to "doctor shop" around until you find one with whom you feel at home/comfortable with, who has the appropriate training, who listens to you and understands your health goals, with whom you can ***work together*** towards achieving those goals and who holds true to the 6 principles of naturopathic medicine!

DOCTORS THAT HOLD TRUE TO THE 6 PRINCIPLES OF NATURAL HEALING
- Doctors of Naturopathic Medicine (N.D. or NMD)
- Doctors of Chiropractic Medicine (D.C.)
- Doctors in Ayurvedic Medicine
- Doctors of Oriental Medicine (D.OM)
- Doctors of Homeopathic Medicine
- Doctors of Medicine (M.D.) who have trained in Functional Medicine or Holistic Medicine.

DO ALL NATUROPATHIC DOCTORS TRAIN THE SAME WAY?
No. Since naturopathic medicine is not yet standardized in the United States, the training level can vary. Some individuals may obtain the title of naturopathic doctor having had as little training as three weeks. Others may have only trained online or in classroom settings but have had no contact with real patients. Some may have even trained for 2-3 years but only in the basic sciences and not with natural therapies.

Since this disparity exists, it is important to research the depth of training of your naturopathic doctor. There are currently only five naturopathic medical schools in the United States that have a four-year standard medical program, including natural therapies, clinical rotations with patients, standardized licensing exams and post-graduation residential programs. The Council of Naturopathic Medical Education accredits these schools and the United States Department of Education finances them. The five schools are:

(1) Bastyr University—*has campuses in Washington state and California.*
(2) National College of Natural Medicine—*Portland, Oregon*
(3) National University of Health Sciences—*Lombard, Illinois*
(4) Southwest College of Naturopathic Medicine (my school)*Tempe, Arizona*
(5) University of Bridgeport—*Bridgeport, Connecticut*

SUPPORT NATUROPATHIC DOCTORS!

If you are interested in supporting Naturopathic Doctors* then please visit the American Association of Naturopathic Physicians (AANP)[23] website and click on the "Advocacy tab". At present, our excellent training is not recognized on a national level. This means that in general, insurance companies do not cover our services. Would you like your insurance company to cover an ND? Then you should read more about section 2706 under the Affordable Care Act (Obama Care) which discusses how states may cover recognized health professionals in your particular state. On the AANP site, you can type 2706 into the search box to see articles about this. Please get involved and help ND licensure so we can help you! Contact your legislators!
You should have a choice for your healthcare! Use your voice!

*Note: naturopathic doctors use the N.D. or NMD (naturopathic medical doctor) after their names. It is up to *the individual* and the state where they are located as to which they use. There is absolutely no difference in training. Any ND/NMD that has attended one of the five U.S. schools at the top will have the same excellent, rigorous training! ☺

OTHER HOLISTIC THERAPISTS

- Acupuncturists
- Herbalists
- Nutritionists
- Craniosacral therapists
- Colon hydro therapists
- Massage therapists
- Mind body medicine therapists/counselors

And many more!

DR. MEGAN'S GEORGIA HEALTH PROFESSIONAL REFERRALS

*If you are in the Atlanta area or ever pass through, **I highly recommend the services** of Nutritionist and Herbalist **Eileen Thorne,**[30] massage therapist **Karen Stephenson,**[31] Chiropractors **Dr. Cheryl Langley,**[48] **Dr. Christopher Scoma**[63] **and Dr. Crystal Jones**[49] and doctor of Oriental Medicine and acupuncturist **Dr. Malcolm Johnson.**[32] Like me, they also have a STRONG passion for helping you naturally heal your body! Their contact information is in the appendix.*

FIND A NATUROPATHIC DOCTOR IN GEORGIA

If you are looking for an ND in Georgia--it does not have to be me although I am pretty cool ☺--then just visit the Georgia Association of Naturopathic Physicians (GANP) website www.ganp.org.[51] Some other great Georgia NDs are:
Dr. Rachel Marynowski,[67] Dr. Winston Cardwell[68]and Dr. Firlande Volcy, ND.[50]

FIND A NATUROPATHIC DOCTOR IN THE UNITED STATES

For general information, or to find an ND in your state, you can go to the American Association of Naturopathic Physicians[23] and click on "find an ND near you". As far as personal referrals are concerned, I have many fantastic naturopathic doctor classmates and colleagues who think like me and love to help people as much as I do!
For example:

- Currently in Charlotte, NORTH CAROLINA **Dr. Melonni Dooley**[52]
- Currently in Dallas, TEXAS **Dr. Blake Gordon**[53]
- Currently in Provo and Draper, UTAH **Dr. Carmel Ferreira**[56]*
- Currently in Tempe, ARIZONA **Dr. L. Evette Ruinard**[57]
- Currently in NEW YORK, **Dr. Mandi Croniser**[58]
- Currently in Phoenix, ARIZONA **Dr. Jose Ventura**[60]*
- Currently in Louisville, KENTUCKY **Dr. Julie Flynn**[28]
- Currently in Phoenix, ARIZONA **Dr. Amanda Roberson**[29]
- Currently in FLORIDA **Dr. Maury**[70]

They speak Spanish! And English of course. I speak Spanish too by the way. ☺

WHAT TYPES OF NONCONVENTIONAL TESTS ARE AVAILABLE?

People often ask me "is there a test to measure the levels of B vitamins or amino acids in my body?" The answer? YES! We can also test for enzymes, minerals or even bad chemicals such as heavy metals like lead or mercury or even do more in depth testing on how well an organ works (like the heart or liver) based on specialty tests for the organ in question.

These specialty tests are rarely done in conventional medicine but in naturopathic medicine or functional medicine, we can test for pretty much ANYTHING in the body. Of course, these tests are more expensive than basic lab work and generally are not covered by insurance so you will have to pay out of your pocket. Nevertheless, it is worth the investment if it helps us get down to the bottom of your problem right? Most of the time a patient cannot order these tests directly, your physician would have to do it. If he or she does not already have an account with these companies, they can open an account. Some of the specialty testing companies such as Life Extension will let you order tests yourself directly.

Listed below are some of my favorite companies along with the main areas they focus on:

DOCTOR'S DATA INC [33]

- **Clinical Microbiology**—looks for bad "bugs" like viruses, bacteria, parasites
- **Environmental Exposure**—heavy metals and chemicals
- **Organ Specific Tests***--they have tests that look at how well Heart, Liver and Digestion cities are working based on the "products" that are supposed to be made in those cities. The Comprehensive Stool Analysis with Parasitology is one such test.

My favorite is the stool analysis test. I have done it for myself and thought it was really cool! ☺ I know, I know. I am NOT NORMAL! Most people find it disgusting to have to catch their poop and send it to a lab.☹ But not me! It was kind of like playing "mud pies" like I did as a child. Of course, it is not mud. Anyway, that is why they call me the "poop doctor"! I used gloves of course. ☺

U.S. BIOTEK [34]

- **Nutritional**—food allergy panels*
- **Immunology**—Candida yeast overgrowth and Celiac disease testing

They can even test for things such as allergies to spices, chemical inhalants, and culture specific foods such as Mexican, Japanese and other Asian foods!

Note: the difference between food sensitivity and a food allergy is that in a food allergy the police/immune system is involved in attacking the food.

Analogy: If your neighbors are playing loud music at midnight, they may disturb your sleep. You have two ways to react:
(1) You are irritated and sleepy, but you do not call the police.
(2) On the other hand, you decide to call the police, which can potentially cause many more problems. The neighbors and the police could have a shootout. Or the neighbors may get angry with you because you called the police and attack YOU once the police are gone. In any case, if the police are called then the situation becomes potentially more dangerous!

The loud irritating music would be the symptom that a food(s) is bothering your system. If you only have symptoms, for example rashes, bloating, indigestion or brain fog but the immune system/police do not actually attack the food that is a food sensitivity. However, if your immune system is actually attacking the food (very bad) then that is a true food allergy. We can only know the difference with testing. You can have symptoms with either case or no symptoms at all. Even without symptoms damage can be done!

LIFE EXTENSION [35]
You can order your own tests from here. This company gives you access to many health articles and you can also call and speak to medical advisors that can explain lab work or other health information to you!
- Basic blood work done in conventional medicine
- Specialty blood work usually not done in conventional medicine

GENOVA DIAGNOSTICS [36]
They do a lot of high tech specialty testing and offer GI and Nutrition university which are videos and online mini classes so that you can learn more about your digestion health!
HOORAY for learning about Digestion health! My specialty!

- **Nutritional**—*VERY* in depth testing on vitamins, enzymes etc.
- **Endocrine**---testing on hormones/messengers/mail carriers
- **Environmental**—mold exposure and heavy metals

LAST RANDOM ADVICE

- **Stay off ladders** unless someone is holding it for you! People are ALWAYS falling from ladders because they were doing work alone and the ladder moved. There is no reason for this.☹

- **Do NOT take other people's prescribed medications**. Period. I do not care if it is your family member with the same disease/issue. This is a great way to mess up your health. I feel like I already said this but it bears repeating.

- **Do not ignore symptoms**! Whether the symptom is new and intense such as strong stomach pain that comes on suddenly and makes you bend into the letter "C" or long but persistent stomach discomfort that is not strong but you have had it for a few days or weeks. Remember the rule of 1's: if you are having a symptom either once a day and or once a week then it is a persistent symptom and you need to get it checked out. If the health professional tells you it is nothing, get a 2nd or 3rd opinion! Your body is SPEAKING to you so listen to it! It is not wise to ignore the "check engine" light in a car and most WISE people will not ignore that light or just hope that it goes away. Most WISE people will take it to the mechanic and demand that the mechanic find the problem. Do not treat your car better than you treat your body. Do not let FEAR of a bad result keep you from investigating a symptom. Remember, the body can restore health!

- **Do not replace your naturopathic doctor's recommendations with the herbal store clerk's suggestions**! These are very nice people to be sure but typically they ARE NOT doctors or health care professionals. Even if by a rare chance there is a healthcare professional working in there, they do not know YOUR health picture! So if your ND/chiropractor/herbalist or person who IS familiar with your health picture recommends a specific product GET THAT! **Example:** Your doctor recommends Milk Thistle for the liver. You ask the clerk for Milk Thistle, and they are out of stock, so the clerk tells you to take Dandelion because it is just as good for the liver. The point is that your health care professional picked the product for you for a specific reason. So if they are out of stock return to your health professional and ask them what you should do.

- Do not **ADD or CHANGE** medications, supplements or their doses without speaking with your main healthcare provider! It is just annoying. ☹ *Analogy: If you were cooking a soup, you would not want someone else adding salt and pepper to the soup without telling you, would you?*

- **Remember this phrase** coined by Sir William Osler 18th century physician **"The organs weep the tears the eyes refuse to shed"**—it means that sometimes we know that there is a problem but we still mentally tell ourselves that everything is fine; and we may *truly* believe it! However, the <u>body</u> can feel stress and will react to the stress whether it is from a positive source of stress--like getting a new job you always wanted--or from a negative source of stress--like being fired from the job that you always wanted. The body KNOWS and FEELS that we are out of balance. The imbalances will usually show up in lab work or imaging but not always.

  Thanks Dr. Nick B. for mentioning this phrase!

- **Do not pop zits/pimples**. You can scar your skin. It is also just gross.☹
- **Prepare your living will**. I know that this is a book about health so it may seem weird to you that I mention this. However, accidents happen and it is important to let your family know what medical treatment(s) you would like if you cannot speak for yourself. In doing so, you avoid having your loved ones fight over what procedures should be done for you. While you are at it, be sure to plan your legal estate as well. It is terrible to witness a family fight over money, so again; at least if you make your wishes known ahead of time it is clear to everyone. Inform your family of your medical and legal wishes as well as your doctor, attorney and a close friend.
- **Wear seatbelts and helmets**! There is no need to be paralyzed or have someone else wipe your bum after you poop because you wanted to be stubborn and not wear one!

- **Wear protective equipment at work**! If they give you masks, earplugs, back braces or whatever USE THEM! Do NOT be a superhero. BE SMART!
- Remember that **health is a journey that is like a marathon, not a sprint**. Some of the older naturopathic doctors who have been in practice for 40, 50 and 60 years say that for every year of illness it can take up to 4 months of actively cleansing/detoxing and consistently getting back in tune with Nature's 9 to truly completely heal the body. Therefore, if you have been sick for 10 years then that math would compute 4 months multiplied by 10 years = 40 months or 3.3 years minimum to get completely healed! Of course, you can see symptoms improving and already begin to feel better within a few days to a few weeks depending on your illness. I do not think that is a hard and fast rule because every individual is different, how people apply themselves to healing is different as are the illnesses themselves; but I would say that I agree largely with that calculation. So do not be in a hurry and instead understand and try to enjoy the journey!

- **Wash your hands before you pick your nose!** That way you do not put dirt/bacteria/viruses into your nose--which can then travel throughout your body. Wash after picking too or use hand sanitizers. The rest of us do not want to touch your boogers/nose slime on door handles.☹
- **Keep cleansing and detoxing!** When do you stop putting gas into a car? NEVER! You put gas into the car for as long as you are using it. Ok, for you smart alecks out there, if you have an electric car you charge it instead of using gas.☺
- **Health is an investment! If you cannot afford to be well, you definitely will not be able to afford being sick!** Medical debt is the number one cause of bankruptcy in the United States! Once your health is poor, it will damage all other areas of your life: work, fun, friends and family! ☹☹☹☹☹☹☹
- **Do not take supplements with high fiber cereals or drinks.** Fiber is a "broom" and will sweep out or pull out the supplements into poop. ☹
- **Natural does not equal safe!** Snake venom comes from snakes which are natural. But snake venom can kill you in seconds to minutes. Natural products CAN harm you! Do not play around with them if you do not know what you are doing. ESPECIALLY if you are on prescribed medications! ☹

- **Do not put Drano/other products** for unblocking clogged sinks into the <u>toilet</u>! It will cause a HUGE poop water problem. I should know. ☹☹

- **You did the crime, now you must do the time**! No whining or complaining or crying about the effort or amount of time it takes to get healthy! You did not get this way overnight! You did not cry after that 6th beer, 3rd piece of cake, 2nd pack of cigarettes, the all night video game fests or partying, the 4th time you yelled at your spouse, the gym membership you never used, not drinking water because it "has no taste", or spending most of your time working and letting life pass you by! Believe me, I am **_NOT_** lecturing you!
I have **_quite_** a bit of "Physician Heal Thyself" that I am working on!
So let us get healthy together! ☺
- _Healthcare_ is something <u>you pay</u> for. _Sick care_ is covered by insurance. Hence, <u>budget</u> to stay healthy**...your life depends on it.**

- **DO NOT BE OVERWHELMED BY ALL THE INFORMATION IN THIS BOOK!**
Pick ONE thing. _JUST ONE!_ Work on that and little by little, you can add more!
You can do this! I did not spend all of this time and energy on this book for you to read the information and then not try to get healthy.☹ If you made it this far in the book then put some of the information to use!
YOU BETTER GET HEALTHY OR ELSE I AM COMING AFTER YOU! ☹☹ Ok, just kidding. I will not come after you, but I could not end the book without at least one threat. ☺

ONE LAST ANALOGY

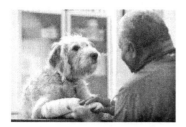

The Guard Dog Analogy

Think of a guard dog, he is your companion by day and by night. He is constantly on the lookout for a potential harm to you, and always does his best for you. Overtime in order to protect you, he has chased away many bad people and listened to you when you needed a soft furry ear. He always keeps your "secrets" and loves you unconditionally! However, recently in a burglary attempt in your home, the burglars injured him while he was trying to defend you! He broke his paw. So now, he is trying to heal. But he is still not 100% healed yet, so if any new trouble does come along, he is not able to run and jump and scare away bad people, because he is still healing. All he can do is bark and try to limp along as best as he can…

Remember, the dog with the broken paw in a cast represents your body and its symptoms *(currently)* and the man represents how we want your mind to view or respond to your body's current state. Think of your body supportively and positively!

Do not look at yourself negatively and say that you have many things wrong with you! You do not have MANY things wrong with you even if you have multiple diagnoses or systems out of balance. You have one main problem and that is that your body has gotten out of tune or balance with Nature's 9 Health Laws! Your body is not working AGAINST you! It has been trying to care for you all this time.

I know that it is hard to see past illness when you are in the middle of it, but **your body has the ability to restore health to itself**--like it does when you get a simple cut on your hand--however, it can get overwhelmed! Therefore, we must first find the cause(s) remove any obstacles to healing, and give the body what it needs such as vitamins, minerals, counseling etc. so that the body can rebuild and restore itself! **You can do this!**

BOOK ALERT: WOO HOO! THE END OF THE BOOK!

Seriously, I am TIRED! I do not have any children, so this is my "baby"! It has been 11 months since I began writing, so this "baby" is 2 months overdue! However, I wanted to make the best "baby" possible! I have tried to put all the information that you typically ask or want to know about when you see me in the office, hallways, bathrooms, parking lots, elevators, stores or other random establishments! I never have enough time to answer your questions so I truly wrote this book FOR YOU the people who I know and for strangers alike! It has been a joy to share my knowledge with you and I hope you will USE it to restore health to your body!

NEWS FLASH: **YOU CAN DO THIS!**

THE END!

P.S. If this **book** was **helpful** to you *PLEASE t*ell your family, friends and coworkers about it! Also, tell the world by ***writing a book review*** *especially* on Amazon, or wherever you bought the book, so that strangers can find the book better!
Help me help others learn about natural medicine and natural healing!
I thank you!

Remember **Health Organizers**[24] working with you to **tidy up your health… *NATURALLY!***
Dr. Megan

APPENDIX: STATISTICS AND REFERENCES

[1] **The top 3 killers** in the U.S. Centers for Disease Control and Prevention. (2014). http://www.CDC.gov.

[2] **Lifestyle and environmental factors** may contribute to 90% of cancers. *The preventable causes of cancer. Molecular Biology of the Cell. 4th Edition. New York: Garland Science; 2002. Cancer is a preventable disease that requires major lifestyle changes. Pharm Res. September 2008; 25(9): 2097-116.*

[3] **Top four life style factors** cause 40-45% of all cancers. *British Journal of Cancer. December 7th Issue. 2007.*

[4] **Dr. Richard Shulze products** and detox programs. http://www.herbdoc.com.

[5] **Amount of protein** in meat. Retrieved from *Live Strong.com. Mar 2014 Erin Coleman R.D. LD, USDA National Nutrient Database.*

[6] **Amount of protein** in eggs. Retrieved from *Live strong.com. Nov 2nd 2013. Lisa Sefcik. Egg Nutrition Center.*

[7] Pesmen, C. (2007). ***5 Operations you don't want to get*** and what to do instead. Retrieved from *http://www.cnn.com/2007/HEALTH/07/27/healthmag.surgery/index.html?iref=newssearch*

[8] **Home fires**. Retrieved from http://www.ready.gov/home-fires.

[9] **Other natural sources of drugs** used in the US: animal, marine or microbial. Retrieved from *http://scholar.lib.vt.edu/theses/available/etd-09062007-000547/unrestricted/Thesis chap 1.pdf*

[10] **70% of U.S. medications** introduced in the past 25 years come from natural products. *Journal of Natural Products. 2007. March 23rd Issue.*

[11] **90 of 121 common U.S. drugs** come from a plant source directly or indirectly. *Benowitz, S. As war on cancer hits 25-year mark, scientists see progress, challenges. Scientist 1996, 10, 1–7.*

[12] **47 % of anticancer drugs** come from natural products or natural product mimics. *Newman, D. J.; Cragg, G. M. Natural products as sources of new drugs over the last 25 years. J. Nat. Prod. 2007, 70, 461–477.*

[13] **Centers for Disease Control** and Prevention. US spent $234 billion on prescription medications in 2008, twice the amount spent in 1999. *Report from National Center for Health Statistics study 2007-2008.*

[14] **Average U.S. dollars spent** on prescription medications per person per year is $985. *Organization for Economic Cooperation and Development. Annual Survey 2013.*

[15] **U.S. health status ranks** 26 of 34 compared to other developed countries, but ranks number 1 in money spent on healthcare. *Organization for Economic Cooperation and Development. Annual Survey 2013.*

[16] **80 % of world uses traditional medicine** as their only/primary form of medicine. *Traditional medicine strategy launched. (WHO News). 2002, 80, 610.*

[17] **Overuse of antibiotics**. *Get smart for health care.* Retrieved from *www.cdc.gov/getsmart/healthcare. May 28, 2014.*

[18] **Nambudripad Allergy Elimination Technique**. http://www.NAET.com.

[19]**Physiotherapy machine** types. Naturopathic Clinical Boards Study Manual 2007 edition Volume 2. Eric Yarnell, ND and Gary Piscopo, ND. Pp. 716-732.

[20] **Prolotherapy** types. http://www.prolotherapy.com.

[21] **Sensory Deprivation/**Flotation Tanks. http://www.FlO2s.com. *this is a local site, so look for float centers in your area.*

[22] **Water filters and Magnetic Therapy**. http://www.nikken.com.

[23] **American Association** of Naturopathic Physicians. http://www.naturopathic.org.

[24] **Dr. Megan's** contact information! *http://www.healthorganizers.net.* *Se Habla Español. Francophone.* Specialty: Digestion. *Poop doctor!*

[25] **United States** Environmental Protection Agency. www.EPA.gov

[26] **Our Toxic World**: A Wake Up Call. Doris J. Rapp, MD. www.drrapp.com

[27] **Environmental Working** Group. www.ewg.org

[28] **Dr. Julie Flynn**. Naturopathic Doctor and Acupuncturist. www.organichealthinstitute.com

[29] **Dr. Amanda Roberson**. Naturopathic Doctor and Educator. www.facebook.com/dramandaroberson and www.deargodblessthismess.com.

[30] **Eileen Thorne**. Nutritionist and Herbalist. SPN Herbs Shoppe. www.spnherbshoppe.com *My current office mate!* ☺

[31] **Karen Stephenson**. Massage therapist. Total Wellness Journey. www.totalwellnessjourney.com. *My current office mate!* ☺

[32] **Dr. Malcolm Johnson**. Doctor of Oriental Medicine and Acupuncturist. Godobe Health Services. Telephone 404.872.2090

[33] **Doctor's Data Inc**. Specialty Laboratory. www.doctorsdata.com.

[34] **U.S. BioTek Laboratories**. www.usbiotek.com.

[35] **Life Extension** supplements and lab work. www.lifeextension.com. 1.800.544.4440

[36] **Genova Diagnostics** Laboratory. www.gdx.net.

[37] **National Health Advisory** health information. www.nationalhealthadvisory.com.

[38] **Bob's Red Mill** healthy flour, cereals and foods. www.bobsredmill.com

[39] **Uncle Sam brand** cereal. www.unclesamcereal.com.

[40] **Wasa brand** crispbread crackers. www.wasa-usa.com.

[41] **Daiya brand** dairy and soy free cheese and foods. www.us.daiyafoods.com.

[42] **Ocho Rios brand** sweet plantain chips. www.myochorios.com.

[43] **Kind brand** fruit and nut bar. www.kindsnacks.com.

[44] **Lotus Wei flower essences** for mental and emotional ills. www.lotuswei.com.

[45] **Oxygen therapies**: Hyperbaric Oxygen Therapy (google to find a local center) and Live o2. www.liveo2.com.

[46] **Organics Happy Family**. Foods for mama, baby and toddlers. www.organicshappyfamily.com.

[47] **Institute of HeartMath**. www.heartmath.org.

[48] **Dr. Cheryl Langley**. Chiropractor. Langley Family Chiropractic. www.langleyfamilychiropractic.com.

[49] **Dr. Crystal Jones**. Chiropractor. Innate Expression Chiro. www.innateexpressionchiro.com.

[50] **Dr. Firlande Volcy**. Naturopathic Doctor. Specialty: Weight Loss. Email: doctorvolcy@gmail.com.

[51] **Georgia Association** of Naturopathic Physicians. www.ganp.org.

[52] **Dr. Melonni Dooley**. Naturopathic Doctor. Solutions for Life Naturally.
www.drdooleynd.com.

[53] **Dr. Blake Gordon**. Naturopathic Doctor and Acupuncturist.
Email: drblakegordonnd@gmail.com.

[54] **Dr. Matthew Baral**. Naturopathic Doctor. Specialty: Pediatrics/child doctor.
www.drmatthewbaral.com.

[55] **Drug-Induced Nutrient Depletion Handbook**, 2nd Edition. 2001.
Ross Pelton, James B. LaValle, Ernest B. Hawkins and Daniel L. Krinsky.

[56] **Dr. Carmel Ferreira**. Naturopathic Doctor and Acupuncturist.
Facebook: search under Dr. Carmel Ferreira, NMD, LAc. *Se Habla Español!*

[57] **Dr. L. Evette Ruinard**. Naturopathic Doctor. Email: drruinard@yahoo.com

[58] **Dr. Mandi Croniser**. Naturopathic Doctor. Email:drmandicroniser@gmail.com

[59] **Evelyn Lumpkin.** Natural Master Chef. Abundant Life Health Association.
www.abundantlifehealthassociation.com.

[60] **Dr. Jose Ventura.** Naturopathic Doctor. Specialty: Family practice with focus on Physical
Medicine. *Se Habla Español !* www.talticpacarizona.com/.

[61] **Dr. Mona Morstein.** Naturopathic Doctor. Specialty: Digestive system and Diabetes.
www.azimsolutions.com/morstein/.

[62] **MannKind Corporation**. Therapeutic products for patients. Inhalable Insulin.
www.mannkindcorp.com/.

[63] **Dr. Christopher Scoma**. Chiropractor. Buckhead Wellness Center.
www.scomahealth.com/.

[64] **Warren Hutson**. Textile/Graphic Designer
Portfolio site:
www.coroflot.com/da_warren
Instagram:
http://instagram.com/da_warren#
Mr. Hutson did a FANTASTIC job bringing my book cover to life! Don't you think? Among his many talents includes a vast knowledge and profound appreciation of the Nike shoe company products. Any Nike company affiliates or executives reading this book should consider him for design of their products!

[65] **Mark Gungor**. Author and Counselor. "Laugh Your Way to a Better Marriage" and other
books and DVDs for singles, teens, men, women, military and family life.
www.markgungor.com. Click on "store"

[66] **Gary Chapman**. Author and Educator. "The 5 Love Languages" and other books for
singles, teens, men, women and social life. www.5lovelanguages.com.

[67] **Dr. Rachel Marynowski.** Naturopathic Doctor. Specialty: Women's and Children's
Health. Intonu Wellness. www.intonuwellness.com.

[68] **Dr. Winston Cardwell.** Naturopathic Doctor and Acupuncturist.
Specialty: Oncology and chronic illness. Atlanta Integrative Medicine.
www.atlantaintegrativemedicine.com.

[69] **Farmburger Restaurants**. High quality hamburgers. www.farmburger.net.

[70] **Dr. Maury.** Naturopathic Doctor. Specialty: Women's Health.
Email: drmaury@equipped4health.com.

[71]**Fresh N Fit Cuisine**. Healthy meals for pickup or delivery. www.freshnfitcuisine.com.
[72]**Plan to Plate**. Grocery shopping; ingredient preparation or meals cooked in home! www.plantoplate.com.
[73]**In Defense of Food: An Eater's Manifesto**. Michael Pollan. 2009.
[74]**Fast Food Nation: the Dark Side of the All-American Meal**. Eric Schlosser. 2001.
[75]**Make An Informed Vaccine Decision for the Health of Your Child: A Parent's Guide to Childhood Shots**. Mayer Eisenstein, MD, JD, MPH with Neil Z. Miller. 2010.
[76]**Childhood Vaccination: Questions All Parents Should Ask**. Tedd Koren, DC. 2004
[77]**Mountain Rose Herbs**. Organic bulk herbs, gourmet spices, loose leaf teas, essential oils, herbal extracts and natural body care ingredients. www.mountainroseherbs.com.

SNEAKY BONUS: DR. MEGAN'S FAVORITE BOOKS!

For the *good* readers who actually look at the back of the book! All of the books listed are actually in my personal library except the first book. It is true we studied all these things in naturopathic medical school but it is great to have other books too! The very first book on hydrotherapy I do not own. I use hydrotherapy books for medical professionals. However, I chose this one for you because I believe it will be easy for you to read and use. Father Sebastian Kneipp was a monk who lived in the 1800's and is one of the fathers of modern hydrotherapy or the use of water in healing! The first herb book on Cayenne is my FAVORITE! The second herb book is great for basic information and the third herb book is more in depth for people who want advanced knowledge. The last two books are ENORMOUS and are not for reading but are reference books for all of the main diseases. Both of them are great! They are very similar so you can just pick one. The Life Extension book has potential lab work to ask your doctor for as well as conventional treatments, natural supplements and nutrition information so that might be a little bit more useful to you. The Prescription for Natural Healing book is probably easier to read though.

- **Healing with Water**: Kneipp Hydrotherapy at Home. Giselle Roeder. 2000.
- A Layman's Guide: **Curing with Cayenne** and its Herbal Partners. Sam Biser. 1999.
- **Herbs for Health and Healing**: A Drug-Free Guide to Prevention and Cure. Kathi Keville with Peter Korn. 1996
- **The Encylopedia of Medicinal Plants**: A Practical Reference Guide to More than 550 Key Medicinal Plants & Their Uses. Andrew Chevallier. 1996.
- **Juice Fasting & Detoxification**: Use the Healing Power of Fresh Juice to Feel Young and Look Great. The Fastest Way to Restore Your Health. Steve Meyerowitz. 2002.
- **Homeopathy 911**: What to Do in an Emergency *Before* Help Arrives. Eileen Nauman with Gail Derin-Kellog. 2000.
- **Acupressure for Common Ailments**. Chris Jarmey and John Tindall. 1991.
- **A Pocket Guide to Aromatherapy**. Kathi Keville. 1996.
- **Prescription for Nutritional Healing**. A Practical A to Z Reference to Drug Free Remedies Using Vitamins, Minerals, Herbs & Food Supplements. Phyllis A. Balch. 2006.
- **Disease Prevention and Treatment**. 130 Evidence- Based Protocols to Combat the Diseases of Aging. Based on *Thousands* of Scientific Articles and the Clinical Experience of Physicians from Around the World. Life Extension. 2013

DR. MEGAN'S FAVORITE BOOKS FOR MEDICAL PROFESSIONALS...*Mainly*

These books are more for healthcare providers: doctors, nurses, nutritionists, therapists ANYONE who is in the "healing arts". However, non-medical professionals can read them too! The first book is my favorite and speaks of the healing power of nature! It was written in the early 1900's and the style of writing and vocabulary may be a little difficult to follow but well worth it! Nature Cure is a guide to the origin of disease and natural treatments and philosophies. The other two books help you understand the interactions between medications and herbs. I really want to encourage the NON MEDICAL PERSON or even a MEDICALLY TRAINED PERSON—untrained in herbs--to be careful when mixing over the counter or prescribed medications with herbs! You can really hurt yourself! ☹ If you want to mix drugs and herbs, seek a healthcare professional who is trained in BOTH drugs and herbs!

- **Nature Cure:** Philosophy & Practice Based on the Unity of Disease & Cure. Dr. Henry Lidlahr, M.D. 2005.
- **A-Z Guide to Drug-Herb-Vitamin Interactions**: Improve Your Health and Avoid Side Effects When Using Common Medications and Natural Supplements Together. Alan R. Gaby, M.D. and the HealthNotes Medical Team. 2006.
- **Herb Contraindications and Drug Interactions**: with Appendices Addressing Specific Conditions and Medicines. Francis Brinker. N.D. 1998.

OH NO! I FORGOT TO MENTION ADDICTIONS! ☹

I am sorry that I forgot! But remember, I am not a professional writer! Anyway, the most common addictions are to alcohol, street/illicit drugs, over the counter or prescribed drugs, pornography, smoking, sex and gambling. Some addictions such as to painkillers may happen after a surgery, car accident or other physical trauma. ***Most*** addictions are caused by an underlying mental or emotional problem(s) from the past or present. When we do not deal with problems in a *good* way, they will come out in a ***bad*** way. ☹ Therefore, the best way to address an addiction is to work with trained individuals to look for the source(s) of the problem. Support the body mentally as well as physically using Nature's 9 Health Laws and natural therapies. Addiction to cigarettes, drugs or alcohol changes how your body works so you will really need professional help with this! Your body will actively MAKE YOU CRAZY for the chemical! There are natural therapies that help with cravings for alcohol, cigarettes or drugs. Create a support network: trained health therapists (you will need a small team), group meetings and individual friends or family who are a POSITIVE support. You may even consider live-in rehab centers. Generally speaking, you will need to ***heal*** from the underlying problem(s) and then change the habits, negative people and way of thinking that put you on the addiction road. This may take weeks, months or years. If you quit and then relapse, try to figure out what your trigger(s) was/were and then remove it/them and start over! It is a process, a journey! However, you ***can*** overcome your addiction!

LET'S GET HEALTHY! WE CAN DO THIS! ☺